KEY STRATEGIES

for

CANCER PREVENTION

*Options to Help You Stay
Healthy and Happy*

HUI XIE-ZUKAUSKAS, PhD

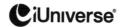

KEY STRATEGIES FOR CANCER PREVENTION OPTIONS TO HELP YOU STAY HEALTHY AND HAPPY

The information, ideas, and suggestions in this book are not intended as a substitute for professional medical advice. Before following any suggestions contained in this book, you should consult your personal physician. Neither the author nor the publisher shall be liable or responsible for any loss or damage allegedly arising as a consequence of your use or application of any information or suggestions in this book.

iUniverse books may be ordered through booksellers or by contacting:

iUniverse
1663 Liberty Drive
Bloomington, IN 47403
www.iuniverse.com
1-800-Authors (1-800-288-4677)

Because of the dynamic nature of the Internet, any web addresses or links contained in this book may have changed since publication and may no longer be valid. The views expressed in this work are solely those of the author and do not necessarily reflect the views of the publisher, and the publisher hereby disclaims any responsibility for them.

Any people depicted in stock imagery provided by Getty Images are models, and such images are being used for illustrative purposes only.
Certain stock imagery © Getty Images.

ISBN: 978-1-5320-8614-4 (sc)
ISBN: 978-1-5320-8613-7 (e)

Library of Congress Control Number: 2019918213

Print information available on the last page.

iUniverse rev. date: 12/23/2019

Medical Disclaimer

The information in this book is not intended to be used as a substitute for any professional/licensed medical advice on diagnosis or treatment of any medical condition. All content, including information, text, and graphics/images, contained herein is for the purposes of public health education and broad help only. Please consult your physician before making any health care decisions about a specific medical condition.

References are provided for informational purposes only. Readers should be aware that any websites or sources listed in this book may change over time, which is beyond the control of the author and publisher.

Contents

Preface

Imagine how you would feel the moment you first hear that a loved one or friend has been diagnosed with cancer. Imagine what it would feel like the moment you first learn that cancer has hit you.

I experienced this moment when I heard of my father's cancer diagnosis. I was in shock, and nothing had prepared me for the news. Three weeks later, my father passed away, and we were devastated. Cancer also took my mother-in-law's life after her battle with the dreaded disease. She had endured surgery and constant pain. Sadly, my father and mother-in-law died of lung cancer, and neither of them smoked tobacco nor drank alcohol throughout their lives.

Whenever I hear that people—friends or strangers—have died from cancer, I understand their suffering and feel very sad. However, I know that I need to do something urgently because feeling pain won't stop cancer.

Deep in my heart, I believe the saying "Prevention is better than cure." In fact, during my medical research, I learned that there are shared factors and features between cardiovascular disease and cancer, the two leading causes of deaths worldwide. Ironically, there was relatively little or lower enthusiasm about preventing cancer more than a decade ago.

Thus, in the wake of our family tragedies from cancer deaths,

I decided to apply my research experience and skills along with my medical background to the challenge of cancer prevention, which is why the website Cancer Prevention Daily was launched in 2009. The website serves as a unique educational resource and has attracted millions of visitors to date, and it has also received lots of positive feedback. The aim is to encourage and empower individuals to live healthy and cancer-preventive lifestyles one step at a time. Together we can make a difference and save lives. Ultimately, we want to save more lives from cancer through a collective effort! Although I provide scientific evidence-based knowledge, refreshing insights, and cost-effective strategies or advice, I decode the content and communicate in a clear and easily understood way to serve the lay audience better. Thus far, I have been translating science and research into public health actions or measures for more than ten years.

My efforts have certainly gone far beyond the website. I've volunteered at a cancer center, fundraised for fighting cancer, and offered free health consultations.

My long desire to improve human health is what led me to obtain a medical degree in China. Afterwards, the need for new drug therapies inspired me to pursue my Ph.D. in Canada. Since then, my research work has been in the field of cardiovascular pharmacology, vascular biology and physiology. Specifically, I have investigated how blood vessels behave under physiological and pathological conditions such as hypertension, diabetes, stroke, and atherosclerosis, and also how vascular structural and functional alterations occur in order to discover potential cellular targets for developing therapeutics. I am fortunate to have worked with world-leading scientists and achieved many peer-reviewed publications in the field.

I am on a mission to save more lives by enhancing awareness of cancer risk factors in daily life and offering proven strategies or solutions to cancer prevention. By saving millions of lives from cancer, we make the world a better place.

I want to extend my work and effort with this particular goal in mind, and reaching out to more people through this book is one of the ways. Viewing blog articles on focused topics online differs from holding a physical book of your interest and reading it whenever and wherever you desire. Furthermore, my blog articles present novel, diverse and expert perspectives on a wide variety of issues, so now it's time for me to compile a tangible collection with updated information in a systematic way.

Writing a book is hard, especially as a first-timer. I've written and published numerous articles ranging from research papers to health communications; however, writing a book is different from what I thought initially and of course, it requires a lot of work and dedication. Paradoxically, it's a labor of love for me.

I am writing this because I feel privileged to have an opportunity of knowing or engaging with your concerns, confusion or needs, and leading you to better healthy living.

I am writing this because I have powerful knowledge to share and would like more people to embrace the knowledge. I want to empower their actions towards reduced cancer risk and enhanced well-being.

I am also writing this because the world needs more actions to prevent cancer. It's exciting and comforting that new breakthroughs have advanced cancer treatments and cures. However, cancer is still the number-two killer disease in the United States and the world at large—right after heart disease—with nearly ten million cancer deaths in 2018 alone.

To those of you who feel powerless about cancer, I'm holding each of your hands and walking down a bright path with you because the process is available and progress is attainable.

To those who want to prevent cancer but are at a loss about

how to do so, I'm here for you as a caring and sound adviser to guide you through your challenges.

I'm also giving you a high five and an enthusiastic cheer to those who have lived by healthy lifestyles so far! Keep it up. Nevertheless, this book may benefit you even more.

Finally, I have an enduring message. If you take preventive measures and live a healthy lifestyle, you are on track to have a healthy heart and a healthy body that will most likely remain cancer-free, and you will have a healthier, happier, and longer life.

I say this because my unique combination of medical background, research expertise and dynamic experience have helped me gain valuable insights into what cancer and cardiovascular disease have in common and how to prevent these chronic illnesses altogether.

Introduction

It was a short time after three in the morning on July 28, 1976. I woke up from a deep sleep because of a shockingly loud sound. It was nearly deafening as massive sounds of thunder clapped in the quiet sky along with a heavy downpour, which was subsequently followed by strong and intense shakes. The lights went off. My little sister and I jumped out of bed, held each other's hands, and struggled to move through our room to open the door in the dark, trembling and shaking in fear. As we tried to open the door, we failed, but we kept on trying with our hearts pounding. Our frightening thoughts, our panic, and the horrible vibration were all too forceful for our small, fragile bodies. Amid the noises of falling things, we were also communicating—in our shouting and crying voices—with my parents as they and our younger brother were also trapped inside a different room. The tremors reportedly occurred for just 15 seconds, but we felt like they lasted forever. Eventually, we were able to open the door, and our family was reunited. Stumbling through the fallen objects on the floor, we all escaped from the third floor of the building together without any injury, which was fortunate. This was a magnitude 7.6 earthquake, the historical "Great Tangshan Earthquake" in China.

Elsewhere, turmoil and chaos were widespread—damaged properties, collapsed buildings, debris-covered roads. Some geographic regions had been destroyed with an estimated death toll of more than 300,000.

That was my first big experience of chaos in my life, and the memory has been everlastingly vivid. Cancer is like an earthquake inside a human body, and it takes away life mercilessly. Just like an earthquake, cancer can strike you out of nowhere, and the consequence of both is the same: the loss of millions of lives.

The internal earthquake (i.e., cancer) creates biological chaos in virtually every part of the human body. Cancer damages the building blocks of life and cells themselves in almost all the systems. Cancer corrupts the genetic codes, triggers disordered signals or cellular pathways, overturns normal cells to malignancy, tears down organs in the body, and finally wipes out people's lives. In contrast to an earthquake, which crushes life from the outside, cancer can eventually engulf and destroy a person from the inside.

Unlike an earthquake, cancer doesn't occur overnight. It develops over a decade or more.

Almost all of us have been touched by cancer directly or indirectly. Maybe you've been affected through a family member or a friend, or you may have already experienced or sustained this terrifying disease. Whether it is slow or fast-growing, cancer can in time take a terrible toll by causing pain and physical, emotional, and financial loss.

However, here's the good news. Many cancers are preventable! You don't have to be a victim. Countless diagnoses and deaths could have been prevented simply with the right knowledge and the right actions, and that is where I come in.

You can also be among many people living happy and healthy lives, and I will show you how to achieve this. This book is designed to help you take vital precautions, apply established strategies or solutions to prevent cancer, and optimize your well-being.

Losing my father to cancer, the hasty and harsh experience,

made me become more emotionally attached to people with cancer than ever. I better understand and sympathize with what their families are going through; that's one of the reasons why preventing this disease is important to me.

We all know the old wisdom "An ounce of prevention is worth a pound of cure" (from Benjamin Franklin). You have the power of prevention, whether you realize or not. I will exemplify and electrify the power of prevention through educating and sharing the truth (i.e., how many forms of cancer can be prevented).

In my humble opinion, knowing who or what factor is most at risk for cancer does not necessarily translate into knowing what you can do about it. Nevertheless, the fact is surprising and perplexing that many people still don't know enough about various risk factors for cancer, except a few such as smoking and genetics. Therefore, the book provides a full package of knowledge and strategic actions to prevent cancer.

Cancer is a serious global public health concern. Prevention is the best investment for individuals, parents, health care systems, and communities.

The book starts by addressing how cancer risk factors (mainly modifiable ones) exist and influence our daily lives before it highlights the roles of these risk factors in specific cancer development. I focus primarily on the most common and deadliest cancers. The book ends with extra guides or tips for a healthy and cancer-proof life.

The objective is to inspire you on mindful self-care so that you can have a healthier body and a better life with exciting ideas, more energy, fewer worries, and less illness. And on a larger scale, through preventive measures we can substantially impact the lives of more people so that they aren't diagnosed with and don't die from cancers.

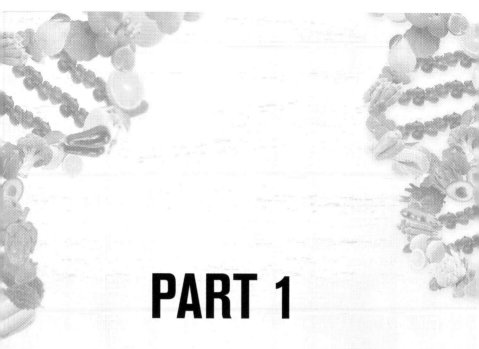

PART 1

Cancer Risk Factors in Daily Life

Basics of Cancer

What is cancer?

Cancer is a generic term for more than a hundred types of diseases mostly developed over time. It can originate in almost every tissue or organ of the body and set off malignancy in anyone at any age.

When cancer cells break away from where they first formed (i.e., primary cancer), invade adjacent tissues, travel through the blood or lymph system, and spread to other distant organs of the body where they form new cancer (i.e., metastatic cancer), this process is called metastasis. Metastasis is the primary cause of cancer mortality.

What causes cancer?

Cancer is caused by genetic mutations—either inherited mutations or acquired ones. Most cancers are caused by a combination of multiple mutations and most mutations occur after birth. Acquired mutations can develop over time through exposure to carcinogens (i.e., cancer-causing substances) or as a consequence of normal metabolism of the cells.

Mutations can convert proto-oncogenes into oncogenes (like the accelerator of a car) or switch tumor suppressor genes (like the brake for a car) to dysfunctional ones.

Proto-oncogene   Mutations →   **Oncogene**

(a gene with the potential to cause cancer)   (a gene in a mutated form, i.e., cancer-causing)

Damages to deoxyribonucleic acid (DNA), the cell's genetic material, can lead to mutations. Then mutated genes contribute to malignancy.[1-3]

A multistage process of transforming normal cells into cancerous ones involves the interactions between internal and external factors. Despite the role of a person's genetic disposition, cancer often develops from a combination of genetic, environmental, and lifestyle factors.

What is your risk for cancer?

A *risk factor* means anything that increases a person's chance of developing a disease, such as cancer.

Some of the known risk factors for cancer are tobacco usage, radiation, some viral or bacterial infections, environmental toxins, age, genetic alteration, and a family history of certain cancers.

Having a risk factor does not necessarily mean you will

develop cancer. Most risk factors do not directly cause cancer given the complex pathogenesis of cancer, but some do. Some people with more than one risk factor never develop this disease, and others seemingly with no known risk factors do. However, nobody is immune to cancer.

In reality, modern society has influenced cancer risk in various ways. Cancer-causing substances exist in the water we drink, the food we eat, the air we breathe, and the things we use in daily life. But what we do on a daily basis can so easily slip into mindless drudgery without us ever grasping the consequences.

Precautious and appropriate measures are crucial to lowering cancer risk, and mounting evidence supports their preventive effects. Based on data from the American Cancer Society, about 42 percent of cancer cases and 45 percent of cancer deaths in the United States could be prevented, primarily by lifestyle change to reduce modifiable risk factors.

Therefore, it is important to know your risk factors because it can help you in various ways. Then you can determine if you need genetic counseling or testing, and you can also make better lifestyle choices to protect yourself from cancer.

Next, let's examine cancer risk factors in daily life one by one and address how to combat them.

Chapter 1

Tobacco Smoking

Smoking, Risk and Consequences

Tobacco smoking is one of the most commonly known risk factors for cancer and the cause of lung cancer. However, damage from smoking to the human body goes far beyond lung cancer. One of three cancer deaths is attributed to smoking. Essentially, smoking is a major—yet modifiable—risk factor for diseases and deaths.

Currently, in the United States, more than 34 million adults still smoke cigarettes, and more than 16 million Americans live with a smoking-related disease. Smoking causes more than 480,000 deaths or one in five deaths each year.[4] A quote (by unknown) says, "One thousand Americans stop smoking every day—by dying," and this mirrors the sad reality.

Smoking can harm almost every organ of your body and destroy you. I'd like to emphasize some smoking-induced adverse health effects and why smoking is actually stressful and can be lethal based on three major types of smoking.

1. There's active or primary smoking by smokers. In this case, smoke is produced from a cigarette butt and directly pulled into the smokers' lungs.
2. There's passive smoking (secondhand smoking or environmental tobacco smoke) inhaled by people around. In this case, smoke is produced from the continued tobacco burns between puffs and exhaled from smokers' lungs within the vicinity.
3. There's thirdhand smoking, which is defined as tobacco-released chemical residues with or without passive/secondhand smoking.

Why is smoking killing you?

Tobacco smoke has been classified as a carcinogen to humans [Group 1]*1 by the International Agency for Research on Cancer (IARC).[5] Each cigarette contains a mixture of more than seven thousand chemicals, including more than seventy well-established carcinogens (i.e., cancer-causing agents). These agents initiate the cellular DNA damage and genetic mutations that ultimately cause cancer.[5, 6]

Convincing evidence demonstrates that tobacco smoking contributes to a wide spectrum of cancers, including cancer of the mouth, pharynx (throat), larynx (voice box), esophagus, lung,

---

*1 When evaluating cancer-causing potential of hundreds of prospective candidates, the IARC places them into the following groups:

- Group 1: Carcinogenic to humans
- Group 2A: Probably carcinogenic to humans
- Group 2B: Possibly carcinogenic to humans
- Group 3: Unclassifiable as to carcinogenicity in humans
- Group 4: Probably not carcinogenic to humans

stomach, colon, rectum, pancreas, liver, kidney, bladder, cervix, ovarian, breast, prostate, and acute myeloid leukemia (AML). Many people know the causal link between smoking and lung cancer. Actually, heart disease is what accounts for the most mortality. As established, smoking can cause cardiovascular diseases because tobacco products make the lumen of blood vessels narrow, reduce blood flow, and elevate blood pressure. They also facilitate fatty plaque buildup in the arteries and the hardening of arteries, leading to hypertension, heart attack, and stroke. Considering that heart disease is the number-one killer in the United States and around the world, the risk of one cigarette a day is still significant.

Cigarette smoking can kill you silently and aggressively, but you don't have to be a victim.

Why is smoking stressful?

Smokers may feel relaxed with cigarettes, but their bodies tell different stories.

With fumes released from a cigarette, there are thousands of chemicals and millions of free radicals, including many carcinogens. They certainly put harmful stress on your body. For example, they speed up aging, stir up chronic inflammation, and damage brain cells or structures, which play a vital role in neurodegenerative conditions. So the reality inside indicates that there's cellular oxidative stress, an imbalanced condition where free radicals overwhelm antioxidant defense. Your body is under attack by smoke-initiated oxidative stress.

Furthermore, ever wondered about chronic fatigue syndrome? In part, this is because of an altered immune system via a link to oxidative stress.

Given the enormous health hazards produced by cigarette smoking, your body is basically stressed out!

Avoid secondhand smoking

Lung cancer is the leading cause of cancer death in the United States. A large majority of lung cancer deaths (approximately 90 percent in men and approximately 80 percent in women) are due to smoking. The impact of passive smoking on public health is disturbing. Passive smoking has been linked to a greater risk for cancer. Epidemiological studies show a causal relationship between passive smoking and an increased risk of lung cancer for the wives (non-smokers) having smoking husbands. As a consequence of smoking, genotoxic substances clearly present in indoor air, and mutagenic chemicals can be detected in the urine of passive smokers, an indication of exposure to carcinogens. Apparently, the non-smoking wives have involuntarily inhaled genotoxic agents in polluted air.[7]

Secondhand smoke has many health risks for non-smokers, including (but not limited to)

- lung cancer,
- lung disorders (chronic cough, lung infections, chronic obstructive pulmonary disease or COPD),
- heart disease,
- asthma in children,
- middle ear infections,
- sudden infant death syndrome (SIDS), and
- an increased risk of having a baby with low birth weight among pregnant women who are exposed to secondhand smoke.

Fetuses, infants and children who are still developing remain mostly vulnerable to the negative effects of secondhand smoke. Alarmingly, millions of children are breathing in secondhand smoke in their own homes. Countless babies are exposed to secondhand smoke in their mothers' wombs. Parental smoking hurts their babies' health and children's long-term quality of life. Because maternal smoking during pregnancy drives fetal malnutrition, tobacco exposure in the uterus causes low birth weight and defects in newborns. And the adverse events in early life influence the offspring's later life such as an elevated risk of obesity, diabetes and heart disease in adulthood. Maternal smoking also doubles the risk of sudden infant death syndrome.[8-10] In addition, common health problems in children show an explicit increase in respiratory diseases and minor sicknesses, which is associated with parental smoking during pregnancy and after birth, and with exposure to passive smoking at home or some daycare centers.

To understand how secondhand smoking raises children's risk of future cardiovascular disorders (such as hypertension, hyperlipidemia and heart disease), consider this view. Passive smoking during childhood has been linked to persistent or permanent endothelial dysfunction (i.e., impaired functions of endothelial cells). Endothelial cells are the cells that are lining on the inner surface of blood vessels and in a direct contact with the blood. Endothelial dysfunction is an initial stage of atherosclerosis and other cardiovascular diseases.

So if you stay smoke-free, it will benefit you and others from becoming less stressed and less ill, and you will likely all live longer.

Alert and caution about thirdhand smoking

Thirdhand smoking refers to chemical residue released from tobacco smoking. It may be described by "the four Rs," referring to *remain, react, reemit,* and *resuspend*.[11, 12] Chemical residues can *remain* on surfaces (walls, doors, floors, carpets, counters, furniture, etc.) and *react* with substances in the environment to create secondary pollutants. All may be *reemitted* through dust in the air and/or *resuspended* long after active smoking has ceased. Here are the key aspects of thirdhand smoking.

The ways or paths of your exposure

Anyone can be exposed to these pollutants by direct contact (e.g., touching contaminated surfaces) and by breathing in pollutants through the air. Outdoor and indoor air intermingle, as outdoor tobacco smoke can enter indoor spaces, and it can adhere to the surfaces or attach to clothes and even to the skin. Moreover, the smoke may circulate throughout the buildings. In addition, you may ingest it unintentionally.

The most susceptible in danger

However, the most vulnerable to the risks of thirdhand smoke are babies and children. First, they usually spend more time indoors. Second, they have age-specific behaviors (e.g., crawling or playing on the carpet, mouthing objects, touching contaminated surfaces, etc.). Third, their developing brains are very susceptible to unusually low levels of toxins, especially nicotine that's commonly present in residue and can harm brain development in children. Thirdhand smoke is often seen in low-income families living in homes or neighborhoods with decades of smoke deposits in the environment.

The adverse health effects

Researchers found that thirdhand smoke exposure (at realistic experimental doses) causes DNA damage in human cell lines. The studies also show that early exposure to thirdhand smoke not only negatively impacts body weight in both male and female mice but also induces persistent changes to immunological parameters in the blood in these mice.[11] We should take precautions about findings from cells and animal models, as adverse health effects on humans still await more studies. However, the American Academy of Pediatricians has recommended limiting children's exposure to thirdhand smoke. And the simplest way to protect children from secondhand or thirdhand smoke exposure is to encourage and support the parents to quit smoking.

Protect our kids from e-Cigarettes

Any form of smoking is harmful, including e-cigarettes. Although they don't burn and release as many carcinogens and chemicals as tobacco smoking does, e-cigarettes contain nicotine, a highly addictive drug, and nicotine addiction can potentially lead people to traditional tobacco smoking.

E-cigarettes are increasingly popular among teenagers, especially with flavors appealing to kids. Thus, they pose health risks for children. Nicotine can harm their brain development. Nicotine has also been implicated in the pathogenesis of cancer and cardiovascular diseases.

The Food and Drug Administration (FDA) has taken steps to prevent the teen vaping epidemic, particularly placing new restrictions on sales of flavored e-cigarettes and kid-friendly varieties. It's important to be aware of the dangers of this drug-delivery system called e-cigarettes and protect our kids.

In summary

Tobacco smoke is a known carcinogen. It is also a preventable risk factor for cancer. The consequences of any smoking are clear:

Tobacco smoke is deadly.

Secondhand smoking is harmful and poisonous.

Thirdhand smoking is invisibly hazardous and equally dangerous.

Despite progress made in stopping smoking and creating a smoke-free environment, we still need a larger and deeper conversation about smoking, especially because the danger of thirdhand smoke and e-cigarette is cloaked in invisibility. The hazards are hidden and long-lasting. There is no safe level of exposure.

What You Need to Do to Quit Smoking

Quitting can reverse smoking's negative impact, and it's never too late to quit. According to the American Heart Association (AHA), smokers who quit between the ages of thirty-five and thirty-nine add six to nine years to their lives, and smokers who quit between the ages of sixty-five and sixty-nine improve their life expectancy by one to four years.

Smokers likely know how bad smoking is for them and others around them, but the problem is that it's hard to quit and many don't know how to quit.

There are numerous methods out there to assist people quit their smoking habit. I summarized a list of tips based on a variety of resources (including the American Cancer Society).

1. You must have the willpower to quit. There is a long list of reasons to quit smoking, ranging from hurting your body and health to the high price you pay financially. You will live longer and stay healthier, and so will your family. However, this one is also worth pondering. Maybe your five-year-old daughter will come home from school

and ask you why you want to kill her and yourself as well.
What a vivid picture of reality!

2. Recognize the consequences of double pollution in our
environments. When you smoke, the cigarette releases
more than seventy known carcinogens into the air and
into your lungs, which is the first pollution. Toxic cigarette
butts on the ground or the shoulders of highways will be
flushed by rain into the gutter or sewer systems, thereby
contaminating our water, which is the second pollution.
How guilty would you feel about such damage?

3. There are *two* common approaches to stop smoking. One
is gradual withdrawal (i.e., cutting down on cigarettes
over time and finally stopping), and the other is "cold
turkey" (i.e., quitting smoking all at once). Choose
whatever works for you; but be prepared for more than
one quitting attempts.

4. Set a firm quit date. Just like working toward a project's
deadline, make sure not to delay it. This date should be no
longer than four weeks from the time you begin cutting
down seriously. (Set yourself free!)

5. Plan strategically. Understand your own smoking
patterns, resist urges or cravings to smoke, and avoid
smoking triggers by focusing on alternative activities to
smoking. You may pick up a substitute item or action
such as chewing a healthy snack or taking a walk instead.
Manage your lifestyle to reduce stress and limit weight
gain. Combine this with a healthy diet, and drink a lot
of water. All will help you handle any setbacks after
quitting.

6. Be patient and persistent. Smoking is addictive, yet you
can succeed in breaking free from this life-threatening
habit if you stick with your resolution.

7. Exercise or actively engage in physical activity. It can make a big difference not only in quitting smoking but also in your general well-being. Pick several activities you enjoy, and rotate them to keep you from boredom.

8. Use nicotine replacement therapy, and/or get prescribed bupropion or varenicline to help. It's important to check with your doctor whether these medications are right for you first. These medicines are safe and effective for most people, and they're available as gum, lozenges, skin patches, nasal sprays, or inhalers.

9. Seek help from professionals and other resources, including books, videotapes, audiotapes, and programs or workshops designed to assist you with quitting. It's always a good idea to check with a health care professional if you are considering quitting. Guidance and support from your physician can be a proven way to better your chances of quitting. You can benefit from a review of your personal health history, reasons to quit that you might not have thought of, tips and follow-up assistance, and new methods.

10. Have defensive strategies for potential problems. One problem is that many people begin to smoke more and not less if they start having cravings. Well, before lighting up another one, how about getting out your calculator to see how tobacco companies have manipulated you and millions of others in health and financial costs? (one-pack-per-day smoking habit costs more than $450 per year if you buy packs that only cost $1.25.)

11. Get support from others, including your family, friends, and co-workers who don't smoke. Support groups are also your allies, and you may team up with a quitting buddy. Telephone counseling programs or one-on-one counseling

may work for you too. Remember that you don't have to go it alone.

12. Join a local or an online chat group for quitting smoking. Make sure to go for some reliable and helpful sources. Be cautious about the internet. Be skeptical about any *guarantees* that you'll quit smoking.

13. Take special measures. Particularly pregnant women, nursing mothers, and individuals under the age of 18 should get medical advice before using any kind of nicotine replacement therapy, whether bupropion or varenicline.

14. Try other alternative therapies. These methods include acupuncture, hypnosis, and herbal and homeopathic remedies; however, their effectiveness is controversial. Do your diligent research before you invest any effort and money in any of them.

15. Reward yourself because you won the battle to fight addiction! After quitting, go for your favorite treats from time to time, or have a party to celebrate your new birthday or another milestone on your life journey. You and others will be proud of what you have done for yourself and your loved ones.

Nothing worked? Yes, you still can quit as long as you resolve to do so! Knowledge is power, and power comes through action. In contrast to costly smoking, knowledge is free and available from many resources. Continue seeking help and strengthen or fine-tune your strategy to create your own workable techniques and eventually, tell your own inspirational story!

Chapter 2

Excessive Alcohol Consumption

Alcohol Consumption and Cancer Risk

Alcohol plays a significant role in many people's lives. There are many excuses for alcohol intake. Relaxing from a stressful day, holiday or social drinking, and youth partying are just a few. But indulging in just one more is often not far from chronic obsession.

On the other hand, alcohol is an established and modifiable risk factor for cancer. Excessive alcohol consumption is also a leading factor for several chronic diseases and mortality.

To use alcohol wisely, it's important to know some facts that are often hidden.

Acetaldehyde, the principal metabolite of alcohol, and ethanol (the ingredient in all alcoholic beverages) have been classified as carcinogens to humans [Group 1] by the IARC.[13] Substantial evidence shows a clear association between alcohol and cancer. Heavy alcohol intake has been linked to several malignancies— oral cavity, pharynx, larynx, esophagus, stomach, colorectal, liver, and female breast cancer.[14,15]

Other harmful effects of heavy alcohol drinking

Excessive alcohol intake contributes to other chronic diseases from liver damage to cardiovascular diseases.[16] For instance, alcohol is known to affect the genes associated with high blood pressure and trigger oxidative stress that injures the inner lining of blood vessels, which subsequently switches on hormonal pathways that elevate blood pressure.

Ways by which excess alcohol consumption causes cancer

How alcohol causes cancer is not definitely clear, but proposed mechanisms include the following: [13-15, 17]

- Alcohol is metabolized to acetaldehyde. This carcinogen facilitates cancer development by either producing more genes that drive cancer growth or slowing down the DNA repair that maintains cell integrity.
- Alcohol-derived endogenous metabolite (i.e., acetaldehyde) can cause DNA damage (e.g., breaking DNA double-strands), and the damage can accumulate due to limited DNA-repair for it. In essence, alcohol intake may lead to permanent DNA damage.
- Alcohol suppresses the immune function, especially cancer surveillance, consequently allowing cancer development.
- Alcohol increases the production of reactive oxygen species (ROS), and drinking heavily can drive chronic inflammation.
- Alcohol raises estrogen levels in women, and excessive estrogen increases the risk for breast cancer as a result of altered biological pathways and carcinogenic metabolites.
- Alcohol causes nutritional deficiencies.

- Alcohol acts as a solvent for carcinogens in tobacco, which explains why alcohol with smoking together is a deadly combination.

How much alcohol is safe, and how much constitutes abuse?

Based on the National Cancer Institute's definition, moderate use implies no more than two alcoholic beverages per day. It can be argued that light to moderate alcohol consumption has been demonstrated to benefit cardiovascular health. Then again, strong evidence from humans also shows that even moderate alcohol consumption is linked to an increased risk of breast cancer in women. Women are more sensitive to alcohol damage than men. Why? First, women have less water in their bodies, and hence, the concentration of alcohol is higher in them than men when given the same amount to drink. Secondly, women have lower levels of enzymes that metabolize alcohol, leaving carcinogenic metabolites, particularly acetaldehyde to linger around the body. The metabolism of alcohol can vary individually, and harm could be done even if there is no bodily warning.

All types of alcoholic beverages are associated with an increased risk of developing alcohol-related cancer. Any amount of alcohol consumption increases the risk and the level of risk increases in proportion to the amount of consumption. Because of this, the best solution is not to drink alcohol at all. As an expert concluded, "Current evidence does not identify a generally safe threshold."[18]

Five essential facts about alcohol for sum-up

1. Through its metabolite acetaldehyde, alcohol is a carcinogen to humans.
2. Chronic alcohol consumption is closely linked to several types of cancer.

3. Alcohol is a significant risk factor for breast cancer, increasing the risk by 10 percent for each drink consumed per day.
4. Women become more quickly intoxicated than men when drinking the same amount of alcohol.
5. The good news is that *alcohol consumption is a modifiable risk factor for cancer*, and it's in your power to control it.

The bottom line is that scientific evidence supports a causal link between alcohol and cancer in a dose-dependent manner. Particularly, cancer risk increases with any alcohol drinking, and there is no safe level of consumption. So avoid or limit alcohol consumption in order to reduce the risk for cancer.

Everybody knows the consequences of drunk driving. Remember not to drink alcohol and use a scooter either!

Chapter 3

Poor Diet

One of the modifiable risk factors for cancer is poor diet. So it's important to examine food quality and hidden carcinogens in the following categories:

1. Processed and red meats
2. High-fat but low fiber foods
3. High-sugar foods
4. High-salt foods
5. Canned foods

Processed and Red Meats

Meat is a popular food in many cultures. It is rich in protein, minerals such as iron and zinc, and various vitamins, predominately B vitamins. However, its contents and hidden effects on the body might make you pump a brake if you're a meat lover. Especially more chilling is learning that processed meat consumption causes an additional 34,000 worldwide cancer deaths each year.

Processed meat has been classified as a carcinogen to humans [Group 1], and red meat is categorized as "probably carcinogenic to humans" [Group 2A] by the IARC.[19]

Processed meats

Processed meat is defined as products usually made of red meats that are cured, salted, or smoked (e.g., ham, bacon, hot dogs, sausages, and deli meats) in order to improve preservation and enhance the color or taste of the food. The products often contain a large amount of minced fatty tissues.

So how do processed meats increase cancer risk? Here is mechanistic evidence.

- Heme iron in red meat reacts with nitrates/nitrites in meat processing to form carcinogenic N-nitroso-compounds (NOC).
- Meat processing can produce carcinogenic chemicals, including NOC, polycyclic aromatic hydrocarbons (PAH), and heterocyclic aromatic amines (HCA).
- Processed meats also contain preservatives (i.e., nitrates or nitrites added and subsequent formation of nitrosamines). Long-term consumption of nitrosamines containing foods (e.g., pickles, bacon, salted fish, etc.) may develop stomach and colorectal cancer.[19-21]

Red meats

Red meat refers to those mammalian muscle meats such as pork, beef, veal, lamb, and horse, including minced or frozen forms. High ingestion of red meats has been linked to human colorectal cancer.

How do red meats cause cancer? Based on multiple meat and processing components, consider the following:

- Heme iron may damage the lining of the colon in addition to its ability to form carcinogenic compounds.

- High-temperature cooking by pan-frying, deep-frying, grilling or barbecuing also produces known carcinogens such as PAH and HCA.
- Red meat sometimes contains high levels of saturated or animal fat and possibly other factors (e.g., hormones). A diet high in animal fat and saturated fat increases the risk of colon, breast, and prostate cancer.

Therefore, eating a large amount of processed red meat raises your risk of colorectal cancer. Daily intake of 50 grams of processed meat or 100 grams of red meat raises the risk of colorectal cancer by 18 percent over a lifetime.

Based on plentiful research findings, it's recommended that people should limit the consumption of red meat (processed or not) to a pound per week (or less than 50 to 60 grams per day) to lower the risk of colon cancer.[21, 22]

Furthermore, the possible role of food preservatives in cancer risk should be an area of great public interest.

High-Fat and Low-Fiber Foods

Not all fats are bad. In fact, adequate dietary fats are essential for human nutrition and health. However, dietary fat is a fundamental contributor to obesity too. What really matters is the type and amount of fat you eat. So let's go through some details of dietary fat.

Why is dietary fat necessary?

It is an important source of energy. It constitutes lipid composition of cell membrane. It facilitates transport and absorption of fat-soluble vitamins. It makes food taste better. Importantly, acceptable dietary fat serves as a rootstock of calories and nutrients for infants or toddlers during their growth and development.

How much total dietary fat do you need?

As recommended for an adult, your total fats should be limited to 20 to 35 percent of daily calories. Then how does it translate into daily fat intake exactly (in grams)?

For a recommended healthy diet, 2,000 calories are needed for a woman, and 2,500 calories are needed for a man.[23] To calculate daily fat intake, let's use a healthy woman's daily calories as an example.

First, calculate the fat calorie range.

$$2000 \times 20 \text{ percent} = 400 \text{ calories}$$
$$2000 \times 35 \text{ percent} = 700 \text{ calories}$$

Next, calculate fat in grams. One gram of fat equals 9 calories.

$$400 \div 9 = 44 \text{ grams}$$
$$700 \div 9 = 78 \text{ grams}$$

So the recommended daily fat in a diet should be 44 to 78 grams in this case.

Why do types of fats matter? What do you need to know?

To put it simply, there are healthy (unsaturated) fats and unhealthy (saturated and trans) fats. Let's examine them more specifically.

Dietary Fats: The Good, the Bad, and the Ugly

The good fats

The good fats are healthy fats (i.e., monounsaturated and polyunsaturated fats). Good fats meet your body's needs and lower your risks of developing cancer and other chronic diseases.

The good fats can be found in the following dietary sources: olive oil, certain vegetable oils (such as canola, safflower, and corn), avocados, nuts (almonds, walnuts, etc.), fish such as salmon and tuna (rich in omega-3 essential fatty acid), and flaxseed.

But not all good fats are created equal. When choosing good fats, quality is another factor to watch out for. Take an example of omega-3 essential fatty acid; the higher its content, the better.

The bad fats

Saturated fats come from butter, cheese, cream (ice cream too), red meats, poultry skin, whole milk, and solid shortening (i.e., any fat such as butter or other fats used for making pastry or bread), to name just a few sources.

A diet high in bad fats increases your risk for chronic illnesses such as diabetes, heart disease and cancer. The negative health impact is based on the following facts:

- Saturated fats may cause oxidative stress, inflammation, and cancer development.
- Saturated fats enhance the tumor-promoting effect of environmental carcinogens, particularly tobacco.

- Saturated fats damage the blood vessels, leading to atherosclerosis and dementia.
- Overweight and obesity resulting from a high-fat, high-carb diet may trigger a cellular inflammatory cascade, high insulin levels, or insulin resistance, thereby favorably providing growth factors for cancer cells.

In particular, a high intake of animal and saturated fats has been strongly linked to an increased risk for prostate and breast cancer.[24] So there are many reasons to put into consideration about saturated fats in available foods.

The AHA recommends that adults should reduce saturated fact to under 5 to 6 percent of total calories. For somebody taking 2,000 calories a day. That's about 13 grams of saturated fat.

The ugly fats—Trans fats

If you'd rather not keep company with the bad fats, you definitely don't want to be found at the dinner table with the ugly ones. Trans fats are the foes of your health because they drive inflammation and raise the risk for heart disease and cancer.

What are trans fats exactly? Trans fats (trans fatty acids or TFA) are formed through an industrial process called hydrogenation, in which hydrogen is added to liquid vegetable oils to make them more solid. So they are processed fats.

Here is the ugly truth. People may not be aware that they are consuming a good portion of trans fats!

Where do trans fats hide in our foods?

These ugly fats like to hang out at the local fast-food joints or in processed food items. The following are some common foods containing trans fats:

- Margarine
- processed red meats (beef, pork, or lamb, especially as the main dish) or other processed foods
- cookies and crackers
- doughnuts and muffins
- microwave popcorn
- butterfat and shortening
- some frosting and coffee creamers
- white bread
- fast foods (e.g., fried chicken, biscuits, fried fish sandwiches, french fries, frozen pizzas, etc.)
- any foods made with "partially hydrogenated oils" (According to the AHA, biscuits and pastries are likely made with partially hydrogenated oils.)

If you eat out a lot, be cautious about foods at many restaurants since there are no food labels that come with your meal and many restaurants use trans fats. The lack of regulations for labeling restaurant foods could be profitable for the restaurants yet hurtful to your health.

How do trans fats impact our health?

First, trans fats raise total blood cholesterol levels, particularly low-density lipoproteins (LDL, bad cholesterol). Second, trans fats lower the level of high-density lipoproteins (HDL, good cholesterol). Higher LDL and lower HDL can increase a risk of heart disease, the leading killer of men and women in the United States. Third, trans fats may promote chronic inflammation. Chronic inflammation plays a key role in the blockage of blood vessels and in the development of cancer.

Remember that all fat is high in calories. It's considered

hazardous when too much fat consumption contributes to the following serious health problems:

- heart disease
- cancer
- weight gain
- other chronic conditions such as diabetes, osteoporosis, multiple sclerosis, depression, and macular degeneration

How do you avoid them? How do you know if the food contains trans fats?

In addition to the previously mentioned facts about the common sources of trans fats, be careful about the words printed on the food package or nutrition facts label.

Here's how you should interpret such words. "Hydrogenated" or "partially hydrogenated" equals "trans fats." "Shortening" equals "containing trans fats." "Trans Fats: 0 grams" equals "likely and/or actually containing trans fats." Similarly, "Trans Fats: 0 grams" equals "contains less than 1 gram per serving," which means that if a food package contains several servings, you may end up consuming several grams of trans fats.

The problem is that it is hard to evaluate the trans fats content in food items, thereby making consumption difficult to monitor. Do you know what you get from one doughnut at breakfast? You get more than 3 grams of TFA. How about one large serving of french fries? You get more than 5 grams of TFA.

Although the FDA requires trans fats to be listed on the nutrition label, there are no labeling regulations for fast foods or restaurant foods. So foods containing the unhealthy fats can even be advertised as "cholesterol-free" and "cooked with vegetable oil." It's also easy to be fooled as mentioned above or misled by marketing tricks and advertisements that often disguise lies under a thin veneer of facts.

Solutions

Only you can say no to trans fats, which is the most effective solution. When unescapable, limit your trans fats intake to less than 1 percent of your total calories per day as the AHA recommends. This means if you need 2,000 calories a day, you should consume less than 2 grams of trans fats (i.e., less than 20 calories of trans fats).[23]

Whereas dietary cholesterol and saturated fatty acids have been shown to have detrimental effects, monounsaturated and polyunsaturated fatty acids in the diet are different. Particularly, foods that contain plant and oceanic sources of unsaturated fats provide unique health benefits such as lessening inflammation and lowering the risk of cardiovascular disease and cancer. Alternatively, replace saturated and trans fats with unsaturated fats, which is more effective in lowering bad cholesterol levels rather than reducing overall fat consumption.

In summary, your fat intake regime is clear. Avoid trans fats as best as you can. Reduce or replace bad fats. Consume good fats.

Sugar—Sweet in Perspective

Sugar is sneaking into all kinds of our daily foods ranging from coffee, breakfast cereal, bread, and sauces to soda, fruit juice, or flavored drinks to candy, cookies, ice cream, and other desserts.

It is crucial to understand that sugar's effects on the body and your overall health depend on the type of sugar (i.e., natural or refined) and the amount of sugar you are taking.

How bad is it?

The AHA recommends no more than 6 to 9 teaspoons daily intake of added sugar. In reality, one 12-ounce can of regular soda contains 8 teaspoons of sugar, which saturates your daily consumption before counting any extra amount from whatever sources. So the amount does matter.

How many types of sugar are out there?

Sugar can be either natural or added (or both). Added sugars are defined as sugars that are eaten separately at the table or used as ingredients in processed or prepared foods.

In terms of source, sugar can be natural or refined. The natural source comes mostly from fruits, while refined ones come from sugarcane or sugar beets. The sugary plants are then processed to extract the sugar.

But sometimes this can be mistaken. Fructose itself is natural sugar in many fruits and vegetables. So, it's not as bad as many folks think. However, be aware of different forms of fructose in our daily foods. For example, table sugar contains fructose and glucose (50 percent each), but high-fructose corn syrup (HFCS) is actually a sweetener. HFCS is typically added to foods and beverages by the manufactures, and it's found in almost everything (e.g., soda, fruit drinks, cereal, flavored yogurt, baked foods, desserts, and many processed or packaged convenience foods). In addition, it's also creeping into sauces, salad dressings, and other condiments.

Of course, in a plain form, there are artificial sweeteners, which are synthetic chemicals. One of them is aspartame (APM). APM is present in a wide variety of foods, drinks, drugs, and hygiene products. Everybody is probably consuming sweeteners—knowingly or not. Do you know that these sweeteners are frequently used as part of a weight control regime? Whether it's HFCS, refined sugar, APM, or any other sweeteners, the sweets are delightful, but they're not sweet to your well-being at all.

How does sugar impact your health?

It's easy to say, "Sugar is bad for you," but just how bad is it? High sugar consumption can increase the risk of obesity, diabetes, cardiovascular diseases, and cancer in both adults and children because too much sugar can

- alter insulin sensitivity, resulting in elevated blood sugar;
- accumulate fat in the body and accelerate weight gain;
- stimulate inflammation, thereby increasing the risk of heart disease and cancer;
- feed cancer cell growth; and
- contribute to various chronic illnesses, including obesity and bone loss.

Take your favorite drinks as an example. Who hasn't had sugary drinks or fruit juice (sugar-loaded beverage)? These sugar-sweetened beverages promote more storage of visceral fat (so-called belly fat).[25] Visceral fat invites serious health problems that we will cover later in more detail.

How about artificial sweeteners? These are inescapable. Despite its approval by the FDA, carcinogenic potential of APM has been observed. Specifically, each molecule of APM releases a molecule of methanol, which metabolizes into a molecule of formaldehyde. Formaldehyde is a known human carcinogen with no safe level of consumption.[20] In addition, consuming so-called calorie-free sweeteners may still pose an increased risk of obesity and diabetes.

How does sugar become popular and in everywhere?

Sugar-loaded foods are often delicious, and we tend to eat more not only during the holidays but also under stressed conditions. Sugar hidden foods are convenient, inexpensive, and abundant. For example, soft drinks (accounting for 33 percent of total intake) are a major source of added sugar in the American diet nearly twenty years ago.[26] How about now? Moreover, sugar "is in all kinds of places you're not expecting to find it, even foods like ketchup," according to one expert.

In 2015, the World Health Organization (WHO) had reduced its sugar intake recommendations from 10 percent of your daily calorie intake to 5 percent. This recommendation refers to all sugar, whether manually added or naturally occurring.

To put this in a more measurable way, consuming 5 percent daily calorie of sugar would be about 25 grams of sugar intake if an adult needs 2,000 calories a day.

- 5 percent sugar intake equals 100 calories of the 2,000 calories per day.
- And if 4 calories in 1 gram sugar, 100 calories equal 25 grams of sugar.

So how does this translate for you? Adults with a healthy weight (a normal body mass index or normal BMI)[*2] are recommended to have less than 6 teaspoons of sugar per day from added or natural sources, given that 1 teaspoon equals 4 grams.

The WHO also warned the public that much of the sugar consumed today is *hidden* in processed foods that are not usually seen as sweets. This is alarming. Sure, you probably know a can of regular soda contains 32 grams of sugar, equivalent to 8 teaspoons. However, do you realize that a tablespoon of ketchup contains 1 teaspoon of sugar (i.e., 4 grams of sugar)?

How about your frozen pizza? Or how about your cereal, bread, soup, yogurt, and even mayonnaise? They all contain sugar. So it's not just soft drinks, fruit juices, or other sugar-sweetened beverages, desserts, and any foods we think of as sweet, but many other common food items, especially processed ones.

How do you limit sugar intake?

First, know your sources of sugar. Awareness is the key. There are some hidden ingredients with many different names in the foods you're purchasing.

The major sources of added sugars are

- regular soft drinks, sodas, fruit juices, flavored drinks or punches, and sports beverages;
- candy, cakes, cookies, pies, and jams;

[*2] Body mass index (BMI) is a standard measurement of weight relative to height (kg/m^2) as body fatness. Based on the WHO classification for adults, healthy weight (i.e., normal BMI) is defined as a BMI of 18.50 to 24.99 kg/m^2 and a value greater than 25 kg/m^2 indicates the following defined conditions:

- overweight as a BMI of 25.0 to 29.9 kg/m^2
- obesity as a BMI of 30 kg/m^2 or greater
- severe obesity as a BMI of 40 kg/m^2 or greater

- dairy desserts and milk products (ice cream, sweetened yogurt, and sweetened milk);
- grains (bread, cinnamon toast, and honey-nut waffles); and
- processed snacks, bars, and breakfast cereal.

Second, avoid processed or packaged foods, including meats, frozen meals, cheeses, and bread.

Third, avoid sugar-dense beverages. At least limit your intake because added sugar supplies zero nutrients but potential toxins and extra calories, thereby putting harm and extra pounds in your body. There are healthy alternatives, such as water, tea, or soda water with a slice of lemon.

Fourth, avoid artificial sweeteners. Choose healthy alternatives for food tastes or flavors, and try sugar-free items.

Finally, consider your children and look beyond sugar and fat to prevent childhood obesity. Teach your kids to avoid sugary drinks, to limit their intake of sweets, to stay away from table sugar (white and brown), and to eat plenty of fruits and vegetables to ensure their wellness later in life.

In short, high sugar intake can negatively impact your health.

Cutting Sugar for Cancer Prevention

Why is cutting sugar crucial to fighting cancer?

Dietary sugar and food high in carbohydrates are absorbed into blood as glucose via the functions of the gastrointestinal tract. Every cell in our bodies needs glucose as a source of energy.

Cancer cells are no exception. They love sugar because it provides them fuel, and they need high glucose intake because a tumor cannot grow beyond 2 mm in diameter without the formation of new blood vessels (i.e., angiogenesis) to deliver oxygen and nutrients such as sugar. Emerging evidence has shown how increased blood sugar plays a significant role in cancer development and metastasis through complicated mechanisms.

Hallmarks of cancer include accumulated mutations of DNA, increased proliferation, and the invasion and migration of cancerous cells. Higher blood sugar has both direct effects on cancer's cellular events and indirect effects on rewiring cancer-related signaling pathways through other factors.

Noticeably, hyperglycemia, hyperinsulinemia, and inflammation are shared biological changes in both type 2 diabetes and some site-specific cancers, which may explain extensive findings that the diabetic population is at a higher risk for cancers of the pancreas, liver, colon, rectum, stomach, bladder, breast, and endometrium. Diabetes is also associated with other cancers such as esophageal, kidney and leukemia.

Furthermore, too much sugar intake can lead to obesity, and obesity is a significant risk factor for cancer. Obesity is also an independent risk factor for cardiovascular disease and many other common chronic diseases.

Diet models to help you curb sugar intake

There are a variety of ways to lower your sugar intake. In practice, follow healthy dietary models such as the traditional Mediterranean diet or the modern DASH (Dietary Approaches to Stop Hypertension) diet, consume the foods with low blood sugar load (glycemic load), low in saturated fat, sugar and salt, but high in fruits, vegetables and phytonutrient-rich antioxidants, along with limited red meats and refined grains. Strong and consistent evidence has demonstrated that these diets contribute to a reduced risk for cardiovascular disease, some cancers, and age-related chronic diseases.

The bottom line is that cutting back on sugar intake will help you maintain a healthy weight and lower your risk for diabetes, obesity, cardiovascular disease, and cancer.

Salt in Foods

Do you have any idea how much salt you consume every day? Sure, food without salt is boring. Plus, salt is necessary for human health and life itself. At a physiological level, we need a small amount of sodium for fluid balance, muscle contraction, and nerve function. However, dietary salt (or sodium) intake in Americans has reached a startling, potentially pathological level largely because of excessive salt hidden in foods we take every day.

At present, salt intake in the general population is ten times higher than that consumed in the past and at least two times higher than the current recommendation.[27]

What is the link between high salt and organ damage?

It has been well established that high dietary salt increases blood pressure. Do you know that about one in three adults in the United States, as well as one-third of the world's population, have hypertension (i.e., high blood pressure)?

Hypertension is a risk factor and a leading cause of cardiovascular disease, and it's responsible for about 50 percent of deaths from stroke or heart disease. Excess sodium increases blood pressure because it holds extra fluid in the body, and edema develops when fluid retention occurs. Increased blood volume means more work for the heart, creating an extra burden on the heart and more pressure on blood vessels. High sodium levels also increase arterial stiffness. Convincing evidence supports that a reduction in dietary salt intake lowers blood pressure, consequently lowering the incidence of blood pressure-related health problems including cardiovascular disease, heart attack, and stroke. High-salt related detrimental effects go beyond blood pressure and heart problems. The kidneys also have trouble keeping up with the excess sodium in the bloodstream. High salt intake combined with high blood pressure can reduce the kidneys' ability to filter out unwanted toxins, resulting in kidney failure.

Consuming salty or salt-preserved foods has been linked to an increased risk for gastric cancer because too much salt may directly damage the stomach lining and increase endogenous N-nitroso compound formation. Further studies reveal the causal effect of salt intake on stomach cancer particularly among individuals who have been exposed to both Helicobacter pylori infection and a chemical carcinogen. Besides, Chinese style salted fish is a known carcinogen and associated with nasopharyngeal cancer.[20]

Too much salt is damaging, but it's manageable. I helped someone who suffers from atrial fibrillation and had edema on the legs. After following my advice, he simply stopped one thing, specifically eating too much salty potato chips every day, and his edema ceased.

Who are at a high risk for cardiovascular disease and serious health problems related to dietary salt?

If you are older than fifty, an African American, have diabetes and chronic kidney disease, and/or have elevated blood pressure, then you are at risk.

Of course, the criteria do not necessarily mean that everybody else is ruled out. For example, increased blood pressure is the leading preventable risk factor for premature death in the general population of Chinese, where more than 1 million premature deaths and 2 million of cardiovascular deaths were attributable to high blood pressure in 2005.[28]

Added sodium supplies more harms than benefits. Sodium doesn't cause illness alone; however, with multifaceted factors, it plays a role in the development of cardiovascular diseases and some types of cancer. So salt restriction is unquestionably beneficial, and moderation is the key.

A Message in Salt: Packed with Twenty Tips

The good news is that you can control your dietary salt intake and take preventative measures against cardiovascular disease, cancer, and other illnesses.

And here, I'm providing you with the top twenty tips for limiting your salt intake.

1. Know the limit of your daily intake. The current dietary guidelines for Americans recommend less than 2,300 mg a day of sodium intake (approximately 1 teaspoon of table salt) but 1,500 mg a day for those at health risks. In fact, the Centers for Disease Control and Prevention (CDC) suggests that the 1,500 mg recommendation applies to about half of the United States population overall and the majority of adults.

2. Know your body. This is imperative because salt sensitivity varies among humans. Specifically, with excessive salt intake, blood pressure in sensitive individuals may rise anywhere from moderately to dramatically. So hypertension has a salt-sensitive or salt-resistant form.

3. Shop smart. Read the labels and compare foods.

4. Track salt in your foods.

5. Cut down or modify. Have the number of your own intake, and go from there to plan your modification. Cut down on sodium in various ways, whether you purchase foods that are sodium-free, low-sodium, or super-low-sodium.

6. Eat plenty of fruits and vegetables. Whether fresh or frozen, you know for certain that they have no added sodium.

7. Limit added salt whenever possible. Consider this particularly dining at the restaurant.

8. Avoid processed or packaged foods where most salt is hidden.

9. Cook your own food. Doing so allows you to know what's in it. For example, steamed veggies (essentially salt-free), and a spiced dish (either salt-free or salt-reduced).

10. Keep your favorite food but choose sodium-free or sodium-reduced versions.

11. Mix half of your favorite item with half of a sodium-free choice.

12. Choose a low-sodium version of frozen dinner food when necessary.

13. Remove salt from the table. When it's out of sight, it's out of mind.

14. Replace salt with spices and herbs in your cooking or on the table.

15. Make a wise choice by substituting a sodium-loaded order with sodium-reduced one. Or pick an alternative without sacrificing the taste.

16. Replace salty snacks with nutritious dried fruits.

17. Replace salty nuts with unsalted ones.

18. Purchase canned vegetables labeled "no sodium added" or "reduced sodium" as alternatives. Otherwise, rinse the veggies thoroughly to wash out some salt before serving.

19. Drink the low-sodium version of vegetable juice. Even better, make your own fresh veggie juice.

20. Create and share salt-free or salt-reduced recipes. Bring salt-free or salt-reduced dishes to your next potluck so that you help promote public health.

Anatomy of Canned Foods

Do you have a variety of canned foods stocked in your pantry and/or refrigerator? Nowadays the selection of canned foods ranges from drinks, juice, soups, fruits and vegetables to fish, meat, and whole chicken. Yes, canned foods are convenient and inexpensive. However, they pose explicit hazards to your health, including increasing your risk of cancer since there's more than just food in the cans.

Let's take a peek inside the cans.

The chemical Bisphenol A (BPA)

BPA, an endocrine disruptor, has been used for years in can liners. BPA has been linked to serious health problems such as reproductive abnormalities, developmental disorders, diabetes, heart disease, and increased risks for breast and prostate cancer.[29, 30] BPA has been proposed as a potential human carcinogen.[30]

According to Consumer Reports, "The latest tests of canned foods, including soups, juice, tuna, and green beans, have found that almost all of the 19 name-brand foods we tested contain some BPA. ... We even found the chemical in some products in cans that were labeled 'BPA-free.'"

Here is the catch. It's important to know that just because canned food is organic, it doesn't mean it is sold in a BPA-free can. And just because a can is labeled "BPA-free", it doesn't mean it has been proven that no BPA exists in the can or food.

Preservatives and additives

They are used in canned foods to add to a food's shelf life. Butylated hydroxyanisole (BHA) and butylated hydroxytoluene (BHT) are two chemicals widely used as preservatives or stabilizers. So how safe or how risky are they? Both BHA and BHT are toxic to the liver and kidneys. They also pose a risk for certain cancers. BHA is a possible human carcinogen.[31] As a tumor promoter, BHT produces chronic inflammation in animals and may react with other ingested substances, causing the formation of carcinogens.[32]

Processed foods

Processed foods are typically altered from their natural state for convenience and for certain safety reasons. For instance, sodium nitrite is used to preserve the color and flavor of meat products. Processed meats carry nitrates and nitrites. These substances combine with stomach acids and chemicals in foods and then form carcinogens. In addition, food companies also use coal tar products (known carcinogens) for coloring and flavoring.

Regular consumption of processed meats is associated with various types of cancer, including lung, colon, esophagus, and liver cancer as mentioned earlier. High intake of canned processed foods also adversely affects your health.

Other ingredients (such as salt, sugar or refined sugar)

These ingredients are commonly found in canned foods. While these products have not been shown to cause cancer directly, they do increase the risk of obesity. Obesity contributes to 20 percent of cancer deaths in women and 14 percent in men. Furthermore, high intake of salt or refined sugar has been linked to cancer of the breast, upper digestive tract, and other organs.

Because children are much more susceptible to any toxins, it is especially important to make sure the food you feed them and the containers and bottles you use to feed them are safe.

The bottom line is that canned foods are mostly processed foods loaded with salt, sugar, fat, preservatives, and some carcinogens with little nutritional value. The best way to avoid these harmful components and improve nutritional status is to eat fresh food.

Collectively, when it comes to your choice of a healthy diet on your shopping list, follow the principle of ABC. *Avoid* canned food. *Buy* fresh food. *Consider* frozen food.

How to Easily Eat More Cancer-fighting Food

How many vegetables and fruits do you consume each day? Today many people do not meet the minimum recommendation. A few guidelines recommend the consumption of 5 or more servings per day of fruits, vegetables, and legumes to reduce cancer risk and maximize other benefits, including protection against cardiovascular disease, diabetes, stroke, obesity, and cataracts.

Abundant human data and experimental evidence consistently support a protective effect of greater vegetable and fruit consumption against cancers of the stomach, esophagus, colon, lung, oral cavity and pharynx, endometrium, and pancreas.

Here are top six tips to help you eat more veggies and fruits with ease.

1. **Eat more by including them in each meal every day.** You might not choose to consume a larger serving for lunch or dinner, but you can incorporate various vegetables and fruits in every meal during the day, including your snacks.
2. **See more colors.** You know that green vegetables are good. So are tomatoes. Add more colors (e.g., light and dark green, yellow, red, orange, even purple or blue).
3. **Gain variety.** It's great if you consume cruciferous vegetables such as broccoli, cauliflower, brussels sprouts,

cabbage, kale, and bok choy. It would be enormously advantageous if you added allium vegetables. These veggies include onions, scallions, garlic, chives, and leeks, also serving as tasty seasonings. How about enjoying a variety of berries? You can munch on blueberries, blackberries, strawberries, raspberries, cranberries, etc.

4. **Experience something new.** It's like a food or health adventure. Try something different, or explore a fun recipe! The point is to find a way to enjoy nutritious eating for your long-term health.

5. **Go easy.** Nowadays activities or duties are demanding. Life is hectic for almost everyone. To manage time and maintain a healthy lifestyle, eat raw veggies and dried fruits, and stock up on frozen veggies/berries.

6. **Go fresh and fast (flexible or fixed) in hot summer days.** Healthy and delicious dishes don't need to be complicated. You likely appreciate cool, light, fresh dishes on hot summer days. Enjoy something light with green leafy veggies or with watermelon that's sweet and super hydrating. Limit greasy and deep-fried dishes.

Remember to drink a lot of water too!

Chapter 4 ───────────────────────

Sedentary Lifestyle

Physical activities involve the movement of the body, which may include occupational jobs, household chores, and leisure-time hobbies (e.g., biking, hiking, or gardening). However, frequency, intensity, and duration vary greatly among individuals in modern life. Convincing evidence supports an association between a sedentary lifestyle and risk for cancer.[33, 34]

Physically Active, Physically Inactive, or Active Sitting Potato: Where Do You Fit In?

Imagine your day. After eight hours of sleep, you get up and exercise for thirty minutes first thing in the morning. After forty-five minutes of preparing to meet the day and having breakfast, you drive to work for one hour. Then you spend a total of eight and a half hours sitting at your desk, working on a computer before and after lunch, and then you drive back home for an hour. After having dinner for an hour, you watch TV, surf the internet, or read for another three hours or so before bedtime. Then the cycle starts again.

Schematic Illustration 1. Your level of physical activity in your daily cycle

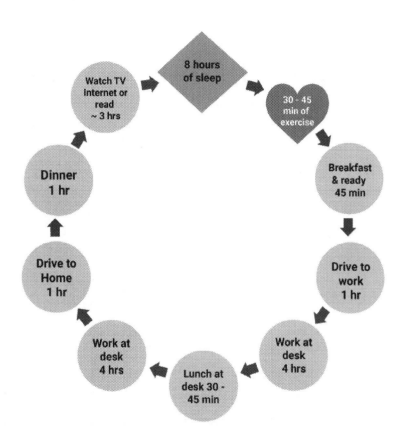

If something like this resembles your schedule/routine, do you realize that you actually spend only about 3 percent of your daily waking hours being physically active? Would the term "active sitting potato" describe you more appropriately? After all, most of your day is spent moving from your driver's seat to the office chair and then to the couch at home.

You are not alone. Recent research shows that about 25 percent of US adults spend approximately 70 percent of their waking hours sitting, 30 percent in light activities, and little or no time in exercise. The modern technologies in our lives—watching TV, using computers, playing video games, surfing the internet, and engaging in social media or chatting over a smartphone—make for a more sedentary lifestyle than at any time in human history. Consequently, we move less and sit more.

Emerging evidence underpins that sedentary behavior (prolonged sitting) is a risk factor for cardiovascular disease, obesity, type 2 diabetes, and some cancers as well as for all-cause mortality. Notably, these health consequences that result from too much sitting can be separated from those that are simply due to the lack of moderate to vigorous physical activity (too little exercise).

What does prolonged sitting do to our bodies?

Well, we know that exercise increases the metabolism of muscles and prevents the loss of muscle mass. It also improves circulation and provides health gains for the heart, blood vessels, and brain. Overall, exercise can enhance your immunity and well-being.

Physical activity not only benefits you by helping you maintain a healthy weight, reducing risk factors such as high blood pressure, hyperlipidemia, obesity and diabetes, and promoting bone health but also offers a blessing to your emotional wellness. It really pays off in the long run.

Positive effects of exercise are indisputable, yet not limited to all the previously outlined. I'd like to emphasize that it reduces your cancer risk too.[34, 35] Sedentary behavior, conversely, has a deleterious effect on the cardiovascular system, hormonal metabolism, and immune functions, and it can lead to developing metabolic syndrome. With prolonged sitting, reduced muscle contractions may result in decreased enzymatic activity for lipoproteins, decreased clearance of triglycerides and/or sugar load, and decreased glucose-stimulated insulin secretion.

Adverse effects of an increasingly sedentary lifestyle over the years include the following:

1. Sitting for extended time can impair or damage your circulation and metabolism that may increase your risk for death regardless of meeting standard exercise recommendations.[23]

2. Prolonged sitting increases the risk of developing several serious illnesses, including heart disease, type 2 diabetes, and various types of cancer.

3. Prolonged sitting or long-lasting sedentary habits elevate your risk for colon, lung, breast, prostate, and endometrial cancer. Importantly, this detrimental association remains even after accounting for time spent on some physical activity.

4. Long-term sitting poses a greater risk for obesity and affects the distribution of body fats, resulting in abdominal obesity (i.e., increased intra-abdominal fat or belly fat).

5. Adverse effects of long-term sitting are not reversible by exercise and other healthy habits.

How does a sedentary lifestyle increase cancer risk?

Accumulating evidence points to a link between sedentary behavior and risk for several cancers. Sedentary behavior is strongly associated with an increased risk for cancers of colon, lung, and endometrium.[33, 34] On the other hand, greater physical activity is associated with a decreased risk for several common cancers including breast, prostate, colon, esophagus, gastric, endometrial, ovarian, bladder, lung, and renal cancer.

Sedentary behavior can cause changes at the cellular and metabolic levels, and the major changes include

1. being overweight or obesity, the latter is viewed as a condition of systemic inflammation and linked to several cancers;
2. altered production of sex hormones, which plays a role in breast and prostate cancer;
3. higher blood sugar, which cancer cells use as fuel to grow and proliferate;
4. lower vitamin D, which may increase the risk for some cancers; and
5. increased chronic inflammation, which can promote some cancers.

Together, these pathophysiological features via multiple ways contribute to the development of cancer and other negative health outcomes.

How to stay away from sedentary behaviors

A wealth of evidence indicates that regular physical activity is linked to a decreased risk for cancer and cancer death. To prevent multiple chronic conditions, current public health recommendations stress that US adults should participate in at least 30 minutes of moderate-intensity exercise each day for 5 days a week or vigorous exercise for 20 minutes each day for 3 days per week. Surprisingly, recent surveys show that more than 50 percent of adults do not meet these physical activity guidelines.

Therefore, I challenge everyone reading this, including myself, to make frequent and purposeful efforts to get out of the chair and engage more in daily activities or movements (i.e., those things we do routinely but are not included in prescriptive exercise guidelines).

Here are some suggestions for getting physically active.

Do it as a priority, and build a routine. Schedule a *move appointment* with yourself and commit to it. Tailor your move appointment to your daily life. Build a routine that works for you so that you can stick with it easily. For some, this could be working out first thing in the morning or stopping at the gym on the way home from work. For others, this could be running or jogging three times a week or breaking thirty minutes of exercise down into a ten-minute walk, a ten-minute yoga, and intentional moves during or throughout the day (such as squat-jumps, stretches, gardening, or other activities). If you consider exercise like a distasteful task, get over it first. It can be as simple as walking, which not only enhances your physical fitness but also stimulates your mental sharpness.

Do it creatively or strategically. If your sitting time dominates, schedule your own standing time or use a standing desk. Other strategies include purposely walking more by parking your car farther away from the stores where you shop or your workplace and using stairways instead of elevators.

Do it more often intentionally. Little bits add up. Make every minute or every move count. Doing house chores, running up and down the stairs, playing with the kids, gardening, doing yoga, walking, or jogging—some or many of these ways of exercising are available to us every day. And you can probably identify even more. The more activities you can engage in each day, the greater the health benefits you can gain.

Do it with others. Take a group lesson, participate in group sport, or walk with company for support and motivation. One of my colleagues used to lead a group walk around the hospital during our lunch break. Also, volunteer opportunities are often physically active.

Do it with variety and novelty. That's another effective way to keep going. Variety offsets boredom, and that's my personal trick. Getting over boredom—trying new things, even by shifting sets or sequences—makes you more likely to stick with your workout.

Do it gradually and consistently. Switching off inactive mode is the first step for fitness. Staying persistently or consistently active can be a challenge, but the reward of your active regime will be enormous. Here's a bright perspective—for sedentary individuals, a modest increase in physical activity combined with avoiding prolonged sitting may help you gain expected and important health values.

Finally, let me cite the wisdom from Lao Tzu, who said, "Do the difficult things while they are easy and do the great things while they are small." He also said, "A journey of a thousand miles must begin with a single step."

These quotes emphasize how great things start off with little steps and how practical an approach can be by breaking a big project into small, easy, and doable tasks for execution. So find your ways to get up off the chair and move more on a daily basis.

Here I'd like to highlight some practical exercises.

Walk to Reduce Your Cancer Risk

A Chinese man who was slim and in so-so health used to ride his bicycle to work as millions of Chinese people do. One day his bicycle was stolen. Although he could easily afford to buy a new bike, he chose to start walking instead. He thought *Walking is good for your health.* He then went to work every day by walking about twenty to twenty-five minutes each way. He also walked to the markets for grocery shopping. No doubt that added extra miles to his routine. A few decades later, he had succeeded in keeping a remarkably good shape. In fact, he eventually outlived many of his friends and colleagues, including those who used to be stronger and healthier than him. His walking routine lasted about thirty years in all before he passed away at the age of eighty-one. He is my father. This real-life story illustrates the long-term benefits from physical activity as simple as walking. Needless to say that walking has been linked to reduced risks of heart disease, diabetes, and other health problems.

Let's talk about how walking is associated with a reduced risk of colon cancer.

Physical inactivity is one of the modifiable risk factors for colon cancer. The American Cancer Society (ACS) recommends that adults should engage in at least 150 minutes per week of moderate-intensity physical activity or 75 minutes per week of vigorous-intensity exercise for cancer prevention.[36] *Going from a couch potato to a gym rat instantly is unrealistic.* A better strategy is to perform small, feasible, immediately executable actions. Walking is a great example.

The good news is that walking at least thirty minutes a day can lower your risk of colon cancer.

Studies from the United States and around the world show that increased physical activity can reduce the risk of developing colon cancer by 30 to 40 percent. In one of these studies, women who walked regularly (twenty to thirty minutes per day or one to two hours each week) had a lower risk of developing colon cancer compared to those who didn't walk at all. Women who exercised at a moderate or vigorous intensity for more than four hours weekly showed a 40 percent lower risk of colon cancer than those who exercised for less than an hour per week.[37] The risk reduces greatly if walking is done routinely for at least ten years.

Other studies demonstrate benefits from walking in a lowered risk of breast and prostate cancer. Furthermore, weekly walking has improved the survivorship of breast, prostate, and colon cancers and decreased cancer mortality.[38] Also, among multiple protective effects of walking is a reduced risk of heart disease, diabetes and other cardiovascular disorders.

To prevent colon cancer, you need to engage in at least moderate physical activity (e.g., walking half an hour a day). All you need are a pair of comfortable shoes, comfy clothes and decent weather. With a positive, can-do attitude, you can manage a routine. In short, walking

- doesn't need any special equipment;
- doesn't require any form of practice;
- is the body's natural form of exercise;
- is for people of virtually all ages and especially practical for middle-aged and older folks;
- can be done anywhere and at any time;
- is simple, feasible, and one of the easiest exercises;
- is safe (but always be wary of traffic); and
- is free.

If walking thirty minutes a day seems too much in the beginning, break it down to small steps. For example, two fifteen-minute or three ten-minute increments can be effective and beneficial, and these might be easy wins as well. You can walk around the neighborhood, in the park, inside a mall or office building, or on a treadmill. Then you can move to a brisk walk.

In summary, for cancer prevention, walk regularly, walk intentionally, and walk lively!

HUI XIE-ZUKAUSKAS, PhD

Ten Simple Ways to Keep Moving at Home

It's natural to stay comfortable and relaxed, particularly at home, unlike working out at a gym. But sometimes home life can become too cozy for folks who really need to get rid of excess calories that would otherwise be stored as fat. And fat accumulated in your body, especially around the waist, can do considerable harm to your health, including increasing your risk for heart disease and cancer.

Here are ten easy ways to help you keep moving at home (or off work).

1. Yoga is simple and doable.
2. Invest in home practical fitness equipment (treadmill, elliptical, or weights).
3. Act on moves beneficial for your balance.
4. Do plank and push-ups on the floor.
5. Take a walk around the neighborhood. Similarly, jump rope or jump squats in the backyard, or run up and down the stairs.
6. Exercise, move around or stretch while watching TV. Likewise, purposefully avoid any prolonged sitting.
7. Dance in the living room with the music.
8. Go gardening. Working at your yard keeps you physically active in various ways.
9. Walk to the local grocery or convenience store instead of driving.
10. Take your kids to the park or the pool, and play with them instead of watching them.

For fun and fitness, learn a new sport that you can play out in the garden or indoors. Sometimes efforts that seem insignificant can actually provide significant rewards.

Several years ago, I had lower back pain. The physical therapist didn't expect the set of exercises that are routinely recommended for such a problem to help my case much. But I gave it a try anyway. Every day after getting home from work, I lay on the carpet doing those exercises the therapist had suggested for about twenty minutes while watching TV. To my surprise and pleasure, my back pain disappeared about three months later and has bothered me very little since then.

Cheering You on to Immune-Beneficial Exercises

Exercises have a profound effect on our immune functions. To further strengthen or rejuvenate your immune system, here are a few types of exercise that could work.

Note that I'm not talking about strenuous physical exercise (e.g., an Ironman race) performed by well-trained athletes. I will examine doable exercises for ordinary folks like you and me. You need to choose types of exercise that are appropriate for your particular situation.

Let's start with *moderate regular exercises.*

You can walk twenty to thirty minutes a day, practice yoga or Pilates, stretch, dance, and even play badminton—all physical activities that can be easily incorporated into your daily life. Moderate, regular physical exercise is associated with many health benefits including lowered blood pressure, reduced weight gain, improved glucose tolerance, better sleep, and increased immunity to fight infection.

A few studies concluded that walking at a forest park (like forest bathing) has increased the activity of human natural killer cells and the level of anticancer proteins, and the result lasted for at least seven days.[39] Because natural killer cells are a part of the immune response to cancer, these findings provide an intriguing perspective despite the small samplings of human subjects in the studies.

Resistance exercise (weight training)

Resistance training ranges from push-ups and squats to weight lifting and weight machines in order to build strength. Maximal resistance exercise increases the acute immune response, which is measured by changes in circulating levels of leukocytes and inflammatory molecules (i.e., cytokines).

To avoid impairing the immune system, allow your body and your immune system the time to recover. For instance, give your muscles 48 to 72 hours to rest between resistance trainings.

Endurance exercise (aerobic/cardio training and repetitive strength training like squats)

Aerobic exercise can stimulate the immune system. At the cellular level, research reveals that acute aerobic exercise greatly enhances a cellular signaling protein (G protein-coupled receptor kinase 2) that is involved in the control of hypertension and heart failure. The protein also regulates an inflammatory response measured by activities of peripheral blood mononuclear cells (e.g., lymphocytes, a critical component of the immune system), which is also stimulated by the aerobic exercise.

Eight weeks of endurance exercise also changed the blood levels of some inflammatory cytokines in a beneficial way in an elderly population and people with certain inflammatory diseases. In contrast, poor exercise capacity in patients even without heart failure is independently associated with the markers of chronic inflammation, which may lead to infections following surgery.

Overall, how exercises improve immune function can be explained in the following ways: First, exercise may facilitate flushing bacteria out of the lungs and airways, which may help prevent upper respiratory tract infections (e.g., colds). Second, exercise may make disease-fighting antibodies and immune system cells circulate faster so that they could detect illnesses earlier. And finally, exercise may reduce the release of stress-related hormones, by which the power of immunity is enhanced and the chance of illness is lowered. One caution to take—prolonged periods of strenuous exercises or overtraining can depress immunity.[40] Thus, the immune system is a complex one, and the benefit of exercise is a matter of delicate balance.

Summation

Regular exercise, physical fitness, and sedentary behaviors are each known to have an impact on cardiovascular health, cancer risk, and total mortality. Despite the fact that too much intense exercise can have a contrary effect on immunity, exercises in various proper forms at all ages are actionable, advantageous, and awesome!

Therefore, keep exercising or getting more physically active one step at a time, one day at a time, and you'll reap the benefits towards transforming your health and life for better.

Chapter 5 ——————————————

Obesity

Obesity becomes a global epidemic. This is beyond a cosmetic issue because obesity is associated with several life-threatening diseases, including heart disease and cancer.

Growing human studies have established that obesity (excess weight) is directly linked to common cancers, such as cancer of the colon, endometrium, breast (postmenopausal), prostate, esophagus, pancreas, gallbladder, and kidney. It is also associated with less common malignancies, such as leukemia, multiple myeloma, and non-Hodgkin lymphoma.[41-43]

Beyond Knowing Obesity Is Bad

As you no doubt know, obesity is a condition of abnormal or excessive fat accumulation that may impair health. The condition results from genetic, behavioral, and environmental factors. Virtually everybody knows that obesity is bad for you, but I want to elaborate further. In particular, I'm going to emphasize *fat*, the adipose tissue in our bodies.

Adipose tissue is not only an inert fat-storage tissue but also an active endocrine organ that's accountable for synthesizing and secreting several hormones and pro- or anti-inflammatory substances ranging from angiotensin, leptin, tumor necrosis factor alpha (TNF-α), and interleukins (ILs) to adiponectin, just to name a few.

Let's take one of them—say angiotensin—as an example to explain the link between obesity and hypertension. Fat tissue has a local renin-angiotensin system, which is well known as an important regulator of blood pressure and a determinant of cardiovascular homeostasis through the action of angiotensin II (Ang II). Being generated from its precursor angiotensinogen (AGT), Ang II causes vasoconstriction, thereby narrowing the lumen of blood vessels and leading to elevated blood pressure.

Compelling evidence indicates that fat-derived AGT contributes to circulating AGT levels and blood pressure regulation.[44] Under normal condition, while most AGT in the blood comes from the liver, AGT produced by fat cells contributes significantly (26 percent) to the circulating pool of AGT. Noticeably, in an obese state, fat mass increases fat-derived AGT, which may become a major source of circulating AGT, thus resulting in stimulated renin-angiotensin system, increased Ang II, and elevated blood pressure. So you can see how obesity is linked to hypertension through fat-derived AGT, one of the underlying mechanisms.

The question is how fat mass is expanded. Well, increased caloric intake, a sedentary lifestyle, and/or various endocrine disorders can all promote fat mass expansion, then cause an increase in AGT gene expression and a higher level of circulating AGT in obesity. Furthermore, with increased fat tissue and circulating AGT, elevated levels of Ang II initiate fat cell growth and thus enlarge fat mass. On the whole, these events result in not only hypertension but also weight gain.

Now let's look at how the presence of fat on various tissues and organs impacts your health.

HUI XIE-ZUKAUSKAS, PhD

Fat on blood vessels

Under physiological conditions, vascular endothelial cells, the inner lining of blood vessels, synthesize and release endothelium-derived nitric oxide (NO) and/or other relaxing factors that induce endothelium-dependent vasodilation, increase blood flow, and play a crucial role in the regulation of blood pressure. We now know that functional changes in blood vessels contribute to the initiation and progression of cardiovascular diseases like atherosclerosis.

How could fat be involved in pathological changes?

Fat tissue around blood vessels can produce inflammation-promoting chemicals or proteins, and these pro-inflammatory factors play a central role in developing vascular dysfunction. Conditions such as hypercholesterolemia or hyperlipidemia can increase the production of reactive oxygen species (ROS, plainly speaking—*free radicals*) in the vascular wall. High levels of ROS can initiate damage to vascular endothelium, rapidly destroy NO and impair endothelium-dependent vasodilation, a condition called *endothelial dysfunction*. Endothelial dysfunction is an early sign of cardiovascular diseases. The abnormality is evident in various disorders such as diabetes, obesity, coronary artery disease, and hypertension.

After feeding mice with a high-fat diet for two weeks, researchers found an increase in pro-inflammatory constituents and a decrease in anti-inflammatory factors in fat tissue around blood vessels (i.e., perivascular fat) but not in fat surrounding abdominal organs (i.e., visceral fat) and under the skin (i.e., subcutaneous fat) in these animals.

High fat mass can also raise your LDL (i.e., bad cholesterol) and blood pressure and trigger insulin resistance, a condition when the cells in your body don't respond well to insulin, resulting in elevated levels of glucose in the blood. Insulin resistance is a key component and/or a driving factor to develop type 2 diabetes. My research has demonstrated that bad cholesterol (especially its oxidized form or Ox-LDL) can cause endothelial dysfunction and reduce blood flow in small brain arteries.[45] Consistent with our findings, mice overexpressing Ox-LDL receptors and on a high-fat diet have impaired endothelium-dependent relaxation in small resistance arteries via decreased vascular NO availability due to extensive ROS formation.[46]

It is worth mentioning that obesity reduces adiponectin, a substance that is secreted from fat tissue and protects blood vessels against endothelial dysfunction. Clinical data show that lower levels of blood adiponectin are correlated to an increased risk of cardiovascular diseases.

What happens with fat inside blood vessels?

You have probably heard about plaque in the arteries, which describes the buildup of cholesterol, fat, calcium, and other substances in the arterial walls. In atherosclerosis, plaques can grow larger because of chronic inflammation, then narrow or completely block the arteries, and they can eventually rupture too. When this takes place, blood clots can travel to the arteries in the vital organs and clog up the lumen of these arteries, thereby blocking blood flow and cutting off the oxygen supply. Consequently, heart attack or stroke can occur depending on a clot's location in the coronary or brain artery.

Collectively, high-fat diet can increase blood cholesterols and body fatness. Fat buildup outside and inside blood vessels together with elevated LDL participate in oxidative stress, chronic inflammation, and endothelial dysfunction; all can lead to the development of cardiovascular diseases.

Fat on visceral organs

What comes to your mind when you hear a reference to belly fat? What I'm specifically talking about is visceral fat (also intra-abdominal fat), the fat stored deeply inside your abdominal cavity and around your organs, unlike subcutaneous fat (under your skin), which is visible and pinchable.

Everybody likely has visceral fat whether knowingly or not. But how much is too much?

Although visceral fat can only be measured by computed tomography (CT) and magnetic resonance imaging (MRI) currently, if you or your loved ones have an overhanging belly and large waist, that's a warning sign of dangerous fat inside. With that said, it doesn't exclude relatively lean (with normal waistline) folks.

So how dangerous is visceral fat exactly?

Visceral fat has deleterious effects on a variety of your organs and their functions. Visceral adipose tissue produces cytokines, a group of small proteins, peptides, and signaling molecules that help the immune system fight diseases, but can also create chronic inflammation and promote tumor growth through multiple biologic mechanisms.

Clearly, visceral fat is linked to amplified inflammation by provoking inflammatory pathways and releasing pro-inflammatory chemicals. Furthermore, through the role of insulin resistance, extra visceral fat may contribute to obesity-associated metabolic diseases and malignancies, leading to an elevated risk of death.[47] This has also been implicated in people who have a normal BMI.

Carrying around excess visceral fat increases a risk for a long list of chronic conditions or diseases,[48] including but not limited to

- coronary artery disease, heart attack, and stroke;
- cancer;
- high blood pressure, high blood cholesterol, and high blood glucose;
- obesity (which makes it hard to lose weight);
- type 2 diabetes (because of insulin resistance);
- dementia and Alzheimer's disease;
- depression and mood problems;
- sleep disorders (e.g., sleep apnea);
- endocrinal and sexual dysfunction; and
- arthritis.

In contrast, curbing visceral fat can be beneficial. For example, after energy intake-restricted weight loss in young and older overweight or obese adults, a reduction in abdominal fat is associated with the improvement in blood flow through increased NO bioavailability.[49]

Here I want to put an emphasis on cancer as cancer's impact on public health is increasingly prevalent. Excess visceral fat is a risk factor for several cancers of the gastrointestinal system, particularly esophageal, stomach, colorectal, pancreatic, liver, and gallbladder cancer. Moreover, there is a causative relationship between excess body fatness and cancers of the breast (post-menopausal), endometrium, ovary, prostate, kidney, thyroid, and multiple myeloma. This is because overloaded adiposity is clearly linked to tissue-derived inflammation as well as alterations in insulin signaling and sexual hormones' pathways, thereby turning normal cells into cancerous ones.[43]

Fat's influence on other vital organs

Just because visceral fat is wrapped around abdominal organs such as the pancreas, liver and kidneys, it doesn't mean that its damaging effects are local. For instance, liver fat may have a direct association with brain aging or brain shrinking. Greater visceral fat is also correlated with a smaller total brain volume, which has been linked to neurodegenerative processes and used as one of the predictors for dementia.[50, 51]

Excessive visceral fat results from a combination of hormonal, dietary, lifestyle (i.e., sedentary), and genetic factors. The more volume of visceral fat tissue you store, the more harm they can supply to your body. So it's clear why any big belly and large waistline are unhealthy.

Obesity and aging

As we get older, we store more visceral fat because changes in body composition occur and comorbidities accumulate. However, hopefully by now, you've come to the realization—if you simply accept that a growing midsection as an unavoidable product of aging, you are ignoring or discounting your health risks.

On issues of aging and obesity, one can't avoid touching on the gut microbiome, the microbial communities inhabiting the human body and containing a diverse array of microbes (in trillions).

The gut microbiota has emerged as a crucial regulator for how our food interacts with our bodies. They modulate how we balance blood sugar levels and how we store fat as well as how we respond to hormones. They play a pivotal role in obesity.[52, 53]

As we age, altered gut microbiota in their composition and metabolites can cause a condition called *dysbiosis*. Science reveals that our gut microbiota undergoes the most prominent changes during infancy and old age, and profoundly, our immune system is also in its weakest and most unstable state during these two critical stages of life, indicating that the gut microbiota and immune function develop hand in hand with age.

Sure enough, with aging, levels of inflammatory mediators in the blood rise, and hence, age-associated chronic inflammation becomes a strong risk factor for morbidity and mortality in elders. It turns out that the gut microbiota may act as invisible yet important players in chronic inflammation.[54]

Aging-associated dysbiosis can promote the intestinal barrier's breakdown, systemic inflammation, and immune dysfunction, which all contribute to the pathogenesis and progression of various illnesses commonly seen in old people such as obesity-related disorders, liver diseases, cardiovascular diseases and cancer. Age-related changes in the gut microbiota have also been associated with some neurological and neurodegenerative disorders as the result of disturbed gut-brain communication.[55]

Together, the gut microbiota can have a potent impact on human health and diseases. But to date, there is no knowledge on *which* gut microbe is doing *what*, *why*, and *how*. Without doubt, we can anticipate learning more soon because of the remarkable pace of scientific research.

Key points on excess body fatness, obesity and cancer risk

If fats deposit where they should not be or more than they should, that will change a physiological condition to a pathological one through the effects of inflammatory cytokines. *Excess body fat is like an inflammation-pumping machine.*

For this reason, any extra fat resulting from both body and diet or presenting in big belly (or larger waistline) poses a hidden hazard. With obesity, people carry not only fat or weight but pain and health consequences. Excess body fatness and obesity contribute substantially to cancer risk.

Obesity is serious regardless of the debate—whether obesity is a disease or a condition. Obesity is just as significant as high blood pressure and high cholesterol. While none of them are actual diseases (but symptoms), all need to be medically treated lest they lead to *diseases.*

Indeed, causes of obesity are multifactorial and complex. However, for some obesity is caused by genetic factors and could be a lifelong condition that needs to be medically treated and individually managed.

Wisdom for Prevention

In most cases, obesity is modifiable and preventable. Lifestyle, diet, and physical activity are key factors to prevent, ease, or slow down obesity even with aging.

So please don't see obesity as a death sentence because it's not.

Nutritional and physical approaches within your control can prevent dangerous fat buildup and thus lower your risk for obesity as well as chronic diseases such as heart disease, diabetes, and cancer.

In addition, getting a good night sleep and reducing stress are also beneficial for a healthy weight because the stress hormone cortisol can increase the amount of visceral fat that your body stores.

Ultimately, consider recruiting your hidden microbial players and keeping them in harmony and happy, which could help your weight control.

Proven and Precise Strategies to Combat Obesity

Weight loss is one of the successful ways to tackle obesity. There are a wide variety of weight loss programs. However, laying out the details of regimes is not only beyond the scope of this book but also likely unproductive for each individual.

Given that obesity is a growing epidemic in the United States and worldwide, weight loss becomes a desire or resolution. Yet weight gain is a big challenge for many people. The novelty of this book is to help you with underlying issues or difficulties. Of significance is to understand how bottlenecks affect weight management.

The bottleneck effect on weight gain

From time to time, most of us have gotten stuck in a traffic jam when driving through so-called bottlenecks. These bottleneck areas often result from the merging of a three-lane to a two-lane highway, a lane closure because of construction, a stop signal, or an accident in heavy traffic. After getting past these, the cars begin to speed up again.

Like traffic bottlenecks, other bottlenecks occur in our lives that affect our health including weight management.

Here I suggest *a new approach* to help you with weight gain or weight regain. You must picture yourself as a problem-solver and apply your willpower to get it done.

The complexity of obesity

I understand your frustrations and struggles, especially given that genetics is nobody's fault. Based on what science tells us, many factors can contribute to weight gain or weight regain after a weight-loss triumph. What I focus on here is behaviors, but I don't throw biology out of the window either.

Visualize this simple model of energy balance: Energy intake equals energy expenditure. Calories in equal calories out. (See the schematic illustration that follows.)

Schematic Illustration 2. How bottleneck effect may influence energy balance

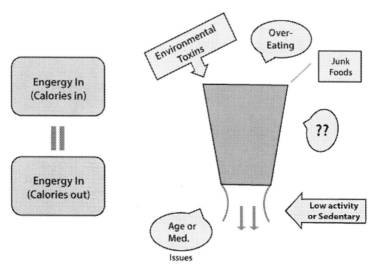

Energy balance   **Energy Imbalance**

Imagine what happens when energy imbalance occurs: Calories in become greater than calories out. Then you gain weight.

Now consider this situation. Suppose you eat healthy and exercise regularly; however, as you age, your pounds start piling up, and you wonder where they came from.

Scientific evidence indicates that many factors may regulate your weight, including

- eating a fat-, sugar-, or salt-rich, red-meat-heavy, or a processed-food-oriented diet;
- overeating (whether out of habit or for emotional comfort);
- sedentary lifestyle;

- exposure to environmental pollutants or chemicals (natural or synthetic);
- intensive stress (from work, finance, or personal life, etc.);
- lack of sleep, particularly obstructive sleep apnea (OSA);
- aging;
- medication(s) you take; and
- chronic conditions.

There's no doubt that each individual's condition is unique. That's how you can be a problem-solver for your weight gain and be a part of the solution.

Where is your bottleneck?

A starting point is to identify the bottleneck for your weight gain or regain. For example, maybe you eat less and move more, but you are in your golden years when your body's hormones change—a *bottleneck*.

Or you may be exposed heavily to environmental chemicals (at work or home) that tilt your body toward getting obese by promoting fat production and reducing metabolic rate—another *bottleneck*.

Or maybe you do have a healthy weight under your watch, but unexpectedly, you then took a drug for some treatment that could alter your metabolism (as many medications do), causing a different kind of *bottleneck*.

You get the idea.

Moreover, what happens if those folks with debilitating pain are unable to exercise as needed despite eating healthy? That's not just a bottleneck. It's more like a funnel clogged at the bottom, leading to limited or minimized energy expenditure. In this case, consult your physician for pain relief and for dealing with the primary or underlying problem(s).

Whatever it is, there is a likelihood that somehow or

somewhere, there is a bottleneck for your weight gain or regain, which is likely relevant to your disrupted energy balance. Finding the bottleneck is certainly helpful, but it's not the final solution. Next, you need to reset or tweak your behaviors and lifestyle based on your body's recalibration to adjust to your situation. Make sure that your solutions are specific, measurable and realistic.

A healthy lifestyle is a journey, not a destination.

Living a healthy lifestyle involves individual choices and behaviors. Modifying your behaviors is within your control. Keep in mind that *every step counts.* For instance, you may eat less, but do you eat right? You need to eat the *right products* (nutrition) in the *right portions.* In addition, beware of not just weight but also how much and where the fat is distributed on your body. Any quick fix for weight loss is not a long-term solution.

Equally important is your perseverance with a balanced diet and regular exercise. Persistence can not only benefit your weight stability but also reduce your risk factors for various chronic illnesses, including heart disease, diabetes, and cancer.

Now act as a problem-solver to discover your bottleneck(s) and tackle the challenge(s) on a weight-management journey. Remember the importance of teamwork too. Always consider your physician's treatment, psychological counseling, and the support of your family and friends.

Best Integrated Strategies to Lose Excess Abdominal Fat

Carrying excessive abdominal fat is very harmful, especially with serious health consequences. Here I share six proven, integrative strategies to lose belly fat and why they work.

1. **Know your risk.**

    Based on current knowledge, what matters more is
    body fat not just body weight. Although BMI remains
    the standard measure to define overweight and obesity,
    BMI does not reflect total fat, especially how the fat is
    distributed. For instance, individuals with a normal BMI
    but a high body fat percentage may undergo a metabolic
    risk (i.e., metabolic abnormality), the condition is now
    defined as normal weight obesity. People with normal
    BMI and abdominal obesity have the highest mortality
    risk compared to those with other patterns of fat deposit.[56]
    Thus, be alert at your warming. A man whose waistline
    measures $\geq$ 40 inches or a woman whose waistline
    measures $\geq$ 35 inches is likely to have excess visceral fat.

2. **Eat a well-balanced diet.**

    Maintain a nutritional diet with caloric restriction,
    particularly eat fiber- and protein-rich, anti-inflammatory
    foods (see a dedicated topic following). Ensure at least
    five to six servings of fresh vegetables and fruits daily—
    essential for dietary fibers. Limit intake of high-fat, high-
    sugar, and high-salt foods. Avoid sugar-dense beverages
    and alcohol. Tracking what and how much you're eating
    is beneficial too.

3. **Exercise, exercise, and exercise.**

    Exercising for thirty minutes each day and five days a week
    as recommended can help burn visceral fat. Types of exercise
    matter too. Do cardio (running, swimming, biking, etc.)
    and strength exercises (weights, push-ups, squats, etc.) to

build endurance. Likewise, the amount and the intensity of exercise make a difference. If possible, find a professional trainer to guide you. To achieve sustained weight loss, both caloric restriction and increased exercise are essential.

If you are eager to speed up the loss of abdominal fat, consider high-intensity interval training (HIIT). Research has shown that HIIT is a time-efficient strategy to improve body composition in various groups or populations. Compared to moderate-intensity continuous training or regular exercises, HIIT significantly reduced the participants' abdominal girth and visceral fat. Overall, this intervention is effective not only in reducing whole body fat and abdominal / visceral fat mass but also in improving vascular health.

4. Manage stress.

Stress plays a role in stocking up excess visceral fat because a stressed body releases a hormone called cortisol (i.e., a stress hormone), which can promote visceral fat accumulation. Elevated blood cortisol levels and increased visceral fat storage are evident in depressed patients.[57] Coupled with the cortisol response, chronic stress-related overeating (particularly calorie-dense foods) also contributes to more visceral fat storage. So stress management with relaxation techniques or tips can be very efficient tools to curtail visceral fat (see details in the chapter on stress).

5. Sleep better.

Too much stress often leads to little sleep. Sleep deprivation sets off what I called a "cortisol crisis" because less sleep causes the release of more cortisol, which can promote fat mass storage through imbalanced energy metabolism and insulin response. Conversely, a reduction in visceral fat can improve your sleep. (See the chapter on sleep for detailed tips.)

6. Rise above tracking weight.

Track your waist and hip circumference. And equally important, track what foods (i.e., the type) and how much (i.e., the quantity) you're eating.

Morbid or severe obesity (i.e., BMI > 40 kg/m^2) deserves medical attention. Because of certain genetic predisposition to obesity and/or genetic variants, changes in fat mass and metabolic response to low-calorie diet may not work for everyone. One of the therapeutic interventions is bariatric surgery (also called metabolic surgery), an effective treatment for obesity to reduce metabolic diseases and enhance the quality of life.

Foods to Prevent Abdominal Obesity and Inflammation

Are you a woman with a waist measurement of more than thirty-five inches or a man with a waist of more than forty inches?

If so, you need to keep engaging in this topic. As discussed previously, abdominal obesity—the accumulation of excess intra-abdominal fat—is grasping our attention to a greater extent, and has been identified as a risk factor of cardiovascular disease and cancer.

Many factors may contribute to increased abdominal fat, including sex hormones, growth hormone, local production of stress hormone, insulin resistance, inflammation and cholesterol levels. Age and genetics are also among various metabolic alterations closely related to this condition. Dietary fructose and fat are involved too. Apparently, you cannot shrink your waist size overnight, and there is no magic pill for it. However, you can simply start with modifying your diet.

How can you do it?

Is there any food that can improve your belly and direct it towards a healthy, active anti-inflammatory way?

Yes. I'd like to highlight eight inflammation-fighting foods.

1. Fish

Yes, you can focus on oily fish (salmon or tuna).

Fatty fish like salmon, tuna, and sardines are not only good proteins but high in omega-3 fatty acids, which help reduce inflammation. To acquire most of these benefits, eat these fish a few times a week, and cook them in healthy ways (grilled or baked, not deep fried, dried, or salted).

2. Healthy fats: olive oil and avocado

Let's face it. Fat adds delicious taste, but not all fats are created equal. So sprinkle olive oil and avocado over your salad, or mix them with your dishes.

3. High-fiber foods: whole grains and oatmeal

A diet study on nearly 90,000 people in 2010 found that those consuming at least 10 grams of fiber daily (especially the kind in whole grains) have waists about three inches smaller than those eating very little fiber.

4. Tomatoes

Tomatoes are a rich source of vitamin C and lycopene, and known to reduce inflammation throughout the body along with supporting the immune system. Cooked tomatoes contain even more available lycopene than raw ones; so does tomato sauce.

5. Kale and other green leafy vegetables

Kale is one of the stars among green leafy veggies, which can make up key components in an anti-inflammatory diet. More than forty-five individual flavonoid antioxidants have been identified in kale, including quercetin and kaempferol. Quercetin noticeably possesses a strong anti-inflammatory property. Besides, kale facilitates the body's detoxification process, which is crucial to flushing out inflammatory substances, such as those built up from processed foods.

6. Nuts and nuts-based fiber bars

Nuts like almonds and walnuts are wonderful snacks as a great source of inflammation-fighting fats and antioxidants. There are so many good things about them. They're rich in fiber, calcium, vitamin E, and alpha-linolenic acid (a type of omega-3 fat).

7. Low-fructose fruits: lemons, prunes, cranberries and other berries

These fruits contain little fructose. Research findings demonstrate that reduction in fructose improves several risk factors associated with cardiovascular disease. In addition, low-fructose diet may be an effective intervention in cancer development.

8. Spices like garlic, ginger, and onions

Garlic and ginger have been used since ancient times as powerful punches to combat inflammation. Garlic can help ward off a range of chronic illnesses, attributing to its antibacterial, antifungal, antiviral, and anti-inflammatory nature. Ginger is rich in antioxidants too. Onions are loaded with antioxidants, particularly quercetin. Many people tend to ignore them, but these foods do add an appreciable taste to your dishes.

Overall, a balanced diet can play an important role in lowering the risk of various cancers and in lessening the hazard of chronic inflammation. A diet with the highlighted foods above can help shrink your waist size. In the long run, it can boost your anti-inflammatory and anticancer capacity.

What else can you do to speed up the progress?

Regular exercises, drinking more water or green tea instead of coke and sugar-sweetened beverages, reducing stress level, and a good night of sleep can all add up to burning your abdominal fat.

Chapter 6 ————————————

Environmental Pollutants and Toxins

When I talked with people about how cancer-causing agents can sneak into the water we drink, the food we eat, the air we breathe, and the stuff we use daily, I often see their expressions turn to agitation mixed with surprise or shock.

Here are some examples of those agents:

- Hexavalent chromium (Cr-6) is a known carcinogen, and it can be ingested from contaminated water or food. Chromate is a very common contaminant in drinking water. How does it creep into our drinking water? There's a simple answer. It's through pollution.
- Chlorinated drinking water is causally associated with the development of bladder, breast, and colon cancer.
- Established carcinogenic foods such as processed meats, red meats, and alcohol (alcoholic beverages) likely are at the top of your mind, at least by now.
- There are other food products relevant to an increased cancer risk, such as burned or charred barbecued food (resulting from known carcinogens PAH and HCA), chips

or potato fries (containing acrylamide, a probable human carcinogen), and heavily salted fish (a carcinogen too).

- Hazardous air pollutants may also be carcinogens. The evident smoking, chloroform, formaldehyde, and naphthalene can be inhaled from indoor environments.

- Most of benzene, acetaldehyde, and 1- and 3-butadiene can be inhaled from sources like automobile exhaust, polluted air, or workplaces.

- Overexposure (occupational or non-occupational) to silica dust, a known carcinogen, is linked to lung and esophagus cancer.

- Household cleaners, stain removers, paints, pesticides, and even personal care products used in everyday life comprise carcinogens. Take carpet cleaner and spot remover as examples. They may contain perchloroethylene (PCE, PERC), a known carcinogen.

- BPA-containing plastics are widely used in food containers, baby bottles, metal food cans, and items such as hygiene products, electronics, CDs, sport equipment, and dental sealants.

The list can go on and on.

Who is at Risk? Who is vulnerable?

Anyone who has been exposed is at risk. Children and elders are the most vulnerable. Occupational workers are also at risk.

Where are environmental pollutants, toxins and carcinogens?

They are present in the following areas:

- industries
- professional settings (e.g., salon, dental office, etc.)
- workplaces
- communities
- homes

In this chapter, I focus on the following areas of environmental influence:

- the top three most dangerous carcinogens at home
- the invisibles from household products in daily life
- air pollution
- the climate crisis

Top Three Cancer Risks at Home

Home sweet home. This American saying might not hold true anymore, especially in terms of health concerns with modern lifestyle. Serious health hazards are present right in the comfort of your home. It's critical to recognize them.

There are three major areas or sources where people can clearly have the exposure to carcinogens; tobacco smoking (including secondhand smoke), radon gas, and chemical toxins (hidden in household and personal care products).

Tobacco smoking is a primary risk factor of lung cancer and responsible for cancers of the bladder, colon, pancreas, and upper digestive system. It releases more than 70 carcinogens. Smoking also aggravates cardiovascular diseases and other health problems as indicated earlier. Individuals who smoke or are exposed to secondhand and thirdhand smoke have a higher risk of suffering from cancer.

While smoking is an obvious danger, radon gas is odorless and colorless, and the worst of all, it's radioactive. Originating from rocks, soil, and dirt, radon can get trapped in houses or buildings and pollute indoor air. Radon is a known carcinogen and listed as the second leading cause of lung cancer after smoking. It is also the number one cause of lung cancer among non-smokers as the Environmental Protection Agency (EPA) estimates. The potential hazards posed by exposure to indoor radon gas is still of great concern worldwide.

Take a tour around the home. Many consumer products—including those we take for granted—make our homes as well as workplaces unsafe. You can find potentially dangerous chemicals (including carcinogens) nearly every room in your home—household cleaners, chemically formulated personal care products, indoor pest control products, plastics, and more. Formaldehyde, a widely used chemical and known carcinogen, can be found in wooden products and furniture, which can also be a source of indoor pollution.

Strikingly, cleaning products are the leading cause of toxic air pollution in our homes, according to the Consumer's Guide to Effective Environmental Choices published by the Union of Concerned Scientists. Ironically, household cleaning products are the most common yet frequently overlooked source of exposure to cancer-causing substances. A smell of freshness and satisfaction from clean settings can mask hazardous chemicals that bring long-term harm to human health.

Therefore, it is crucial to seriously reconsider household cleaning supplies and indoor air quality. Take these three measures to avoid or limit your exposure to indoor air pollutants and reduce your risk of cancer.

1. Stop smoking. Avoid passive smoking, and become aware of thirdhand smoking.
2. Take precaution against radon gas by increasing ventilation and getting your home tested for radon level.
3. Practice chemical-free and carcinogen-free cleaning.

Besides taking control of cancer-causing substances at your home, lifestyle modification is of significance in cancer prevention too. Eat plenty of fruits and vegetables, avoid alcohol intake, limit the use of personal care or cosmetic products, get active and become fit. All these actions will help you keep cancer at bay.

The key takeaway is that just because you cannot see or smell something, it doesn't mean that your homes are toxin-free as carcinogens and chemical pollutants are evidently sneaking into what you use and where you live. So make your home safe and healthier.

The Dirt on Household Cleaners: Hazardous or Beneficial?

What cleaning products do you use to keep your home clean and sparkle? Without realizing it, people have put health hazards in their homes while using many popularly branded cleaners. On top of it, they likely use the spray bottles loaded with some toxic chemicals and disperse them into the air they breathe. With tiny droplets and residue, the risks for allergy, asthma, and cancer are considerably increased.

What are hiding in those cleaning agents?

Toxic ingredients in household cleaning products contain carcinogens in addition to endocrine disrupters and neurotoxins. Several carcinogens that are classified by the IARC are commonly found in household cleaners.

A carpet cleaner or spot remover may contain PCE (also called or tetrachloroethylene), a known carcinogen, and it is also used for dry-cleaning fabrics. A paint stripper may contain methylene chloride, a possible human carcinogen. Mothballs and moth crystals contain either naphthalene or paradichlorobenzene, a possible human carcinogen. Laundry detergents may contain trisodium nitrilotriacetate (NTA), a possible human carcinogen.

Other known carcinogens to humans [Group 1] such as benzene, formaldehyde, vinyl chloride, and carbon tetrachloride [20] are also present in household cleaning products.

The ugly truth is that it often takes years and decades to develop cancer through continual exposure to dangerous chemicals or even possibly long after chronic exposure. It's such a sad aftermath. With the right knowledge, we can control the exposure and avoid the cancer risks discussed here.

What paths do these pollutants or toxins travel?

They can remain on any surface you've cleaned. They can enter your body via inhalation, contact, or possible ingestion.

For a pregnant woman, these pollutants or toxins can migrate through her own body into that of her baby, where they can damage the developing brain or other organs of a fetus. As a result, a baby could be born with a defect or illness.

These poisons can cycle back into your home too. Although you may feel safe after watching the used chemicals disappear down the drain or toilet, it is possible for them to leach back into the tap water systems.

The point is that even if the amounts are tiny and the particles are invisible, these pollutants can build up over time, still may contaminate the water we drink or cook with, shower in or wash our clothes and dishes. So make sure what you're using at home is safe, not just convenient. Think before you pour any chemicals down the drain.

More importantly, take action to protect yourself and your loved ones. Go through your household cleaners—bathroom disinfectants, glass cleaners, drain cleaners, oven cleaners, dish detergents, garden pesticides, paints, paint strippers, stain removers, furniture polish, detergents, degreasers, and even flea powders. Check to see if any toxic and cancerous ingredients are present, and safely eliminate them.

Plastics, Potentials, and Protection

The consumer's usage of many plastic containers and bottles has been linked to cancer risk. Numerous scientific studies have demonstrated that a biologically active chemical BPA is released from polycarbonate bottles into the bottle content after simulated normal use. BPA can leach out into food or water when the plastic item is washed, heated, and/or reused. This impacts adults as well as children.

Other everyday plastic products are not all safe. For example, phthalates (possible human carcinogens and endocrine disruptors) find their ways to food packaging or wraps, toys, vinyl flooring, shower curtains, and medical devices. Beyond plastics, they can be found in the air through vapors or dust contaminated with phthalates.

To protect yourself and family from serious health problems and cancer risks associated with exposure to BPA, phthalates and endocrine disrupting chemicals alike, here are more attainable actions.

First, know your plastics. The number inside the universal recycling symbol (with three chasing arrows) simply represents the type of plastic being used.

Second, become wise with plastics. Sort out what to use and what to avoid. When annual spring-cleaning comes, jump in with inspiration or self-protection, and put some effort into decluttering these potential health hazards.

Finally, protect the safety of others and the earth. There are different kinds of recycling symbols, and not all plastics are recyclable. So make sure to follow the instructions or contact the local municipal authority for proper approaches. Recycle, reuse, and reduce.

Air Pollution as a Carcinogenic Factor

Nowadays when we take a deep breath, we are likely breathing in polluted air.

The sky in the United States is not smoggy, so the air may seem relatively clean. However, there can be many invisible pollutants in the air we breathe, including chemical toxins, radiation, and biological or infectious agents. A variety of pollutants can also emerge in our water and soil.

Air pollution is a mixture of natural and man-made substances in the air, and it's present in outdoor and indoor environment. We humans get exposure to a wide spectrum of air pollutants. Common ones include ozone (O_3), nitrogen dioxide (NO_2), carbon monoxide (CO), sulfur or sulfur dioxide (SO_2), and particulate matter (PM10 and PM2.5). Others are allergens or irritants, smoking and vaping, arsenic, lead, radiation, sun rays, bacteria and viruses, and mold in the surrounding air. Alarmingly, climate change is the result from buildup of greenhouse gases.

The IARC has classified outdoor air pollution as carcinogenic to humans. Overwhelming evidence has pointed to how our environment plays a vital role in public health, including an increased risk for different forms of cancer. The danger of air pollutants lies in the fact that they cause DNA damage, a known and critical event in the development of cancer. Undoubtedly, factors outside the body can change the components and systems inside the body over time.

It is disturbing to learn from some studies conducted in Asia that children in major cities of developing countries have an increased risk for cancer as a result of exposure to genotoxic substances in the air.[58]

Many cancers can be prevented by maintaining an environmental conscience and undergoing lifestyle modification. Making wise choices for our families and communities is vital because we must safeguard not only our own health and our children's well-being but that of future generations too.

Pollutants are all around us, and many of them are man-made. Let's all strive to make every day a clean air day. A healthy earth with a healthy environment promotes healthy living for each and every one of us.

The Climate Crisis Is a Health Crisis

Climate change is not a buzz word or science fiction, but rather it's an urgent crisis based on scientific facts. The United Nations (UN)'s Sustainable Development Goals (SDG 13: Climate Action) calls for the world to "take urgent action to combat climate change and its impact."

So how urgent? And how does climate change affect you?

A plain fact is that greenhouse gases (especially carbon dioxide, CO_2) absorb heat. The climate becomes warmer and warmer because CO_2 has been released into the atmosphere in increasingly faster and larger amounts. This acceleration of the greenhouse effect results from the expansion of fossil fuel burning, livestock farming, deforestation, and other practices over past decades. Basically, these are human activities.

Consequently, we see more and more extreme weather, dangerous heat, rising seas, flooding(s), wildfires, hurricanes, and disasters. These events endanger the beauty and richness of the planet and the harmony of the ecosystem, and they threaten national security (seriously). More alarming, they take not only economic tolls but also tolls on human lives by their severe impact on public health.

We have a window of twelve years to reduce carbon emissions. The well-being of future generations depends on and demands our speedy actions.

Let us focus on exactly how climate change can impact human health.

We know that dangerous storms and subsequent flooding by heavy rains cause more contaminated water, more environmental pollutants, and more disease-spreading pathogens, leading to more human deaths. As the WHO assessed, upsurges in malnutrition, malaria, diarrhea, and heat stress caused by climate change could kill an additional 250,000 people each year by 2030.

We know that warmer regions harbor more disease-carrying insects, and climate change has altered the geographic pattern of these bugs. For example, Lyme disease, an infection spread by tick bites, reached its highest occurrence in 2017, with reported

40,000 cases after steadily growing since 1991. These numbers are based on the CDC's data.

We know that dangerous heat waves and extreme weather patterns cause more psychological distress, depression, and other mental health concerns.

We also know that more water vapor creates a thicker blanket of pollutants—not only warming the earth but producing reduced air quality. Additionally, high temperatures render inert chemicals more volatile and more soluble. Some of the compounds are carcinogenic or possibly carcinogenic, and human exposure to them is cumulative. The more pollutants around, the more asthma, respiratory diseases, diabetes, cardiovascular diseases, and cancer.

All of this is indisputable.

Importantly, we also know that our human activities—ironically, including human convenience—have led to today's *inconvenient truth*. Therefore, each and every one of us has a responsibility to act without delay.

Some people in some demographics might dismiss the urgency of dealing with climate change, thinking it doesn't affect them. It is true that the poor and minorities are often the victims most at risk of suffering from communicable diseases, and among them, the most vulnerable are children. However, climate change affects everyone because it has set off growing incidences of noncommunicable diseases (e.g., heart disease and cancer) in countries around the world.

There are numerous ways to reduce greenhouse gas emissions, and I'd like to share *seven* top ideas for taking greener actions and lifestyle modifications on a daily basis.

1. Bike or walk instead of driving whenever possible to reduce your carbon fingerprint and overcome a sedentary lifestyle.

2. Buy local products to reduce fossil fuel for transportation and greenhouse gas emission, and if it is close to home, walk to the farmers' market. Needless to say that the better quality of food you will likely find there doubles your health benefits.

3. Cut meat consumption, especially red meats, and embrace a plant-based diet. Less meat does not equal no meat. By eating less meat, you help curtail livestock production and coexistent greenhouse emissions while lowering your intake of potentially carcinogenic agents.

4. Recycle, recycle, and recycle. And even better, minimize the use of plastics from water bottles to plastic bags and straws in order to prevent environmental pollution and cut carbon emissions.

5. Reuse items when possible to reduce wastes in landfills. Reuse grocery/shopping bags, and reuse other household products or personal items after repairing. You may also donate useful items to charitable organizations.

6. Unplug electronic devices, turn off TVs, and switch off lights when not in use to curtail carbon dioxide emission by utilizing less electricity and preserving more natural resources, particularly in the evening. Doing so will also promote a good night's sleep.

7. Plant a garden or a tree around the house if you haven't yet to offset the greenhouse effect and global warming as plants and trees take in carbon dioxide. Plus gardening keeps you physically active.

It all comes down to behavioral change, and at times it takes giving up some convenience. You have a choice to act on one thing or all the above, and certainly, you can go further.

I challenge you to make a thoughtful resolution or update

your New Year's resolutions and contribute personal effort to combating global warming.

Imagine what changes that effort will bring to the world when it's multiplied many times.

Again, climate change and health impact go hand in hand. So let's save the planet, save the world, and save lives!

How Can Climate Change Impact Cancer Risk?

Much of the talk in the summer months is about a heat wave. People ask, "Are you cooked? Are you baked?"

Yes, massive, harsh, and dangerous heat waves that hit most regions of the country are certainly unwelcomed and unexpected in its increasing intensity, frequency, and duration. Sure, Mother Nature is something to blame, but climate change and consequential global warming cannot be ignored.

Global warming is no longer a theory. It's a reality. A warming planet undoubtedly plays a role in human lives and health.

Therefore, I'd like to weigh in an issue seemingly less visible yet closely related. A more specific question should be addressed. Is there a connection between climate change and cancer development? If so, what is the connection?

As an alarming and disturbing note, climate change poses the biggest threat to public health in the twenty-first century.[60] Solid science has told us so. My focus here is to explain how climate change directly and indirectly influences the risk of cancer in six ways.

1. It increases our exposure to toxic chemicals by heavy and long-lasting rainfalls or floods. Global warming followed by excessive rainfalls wash toxic chemicals into the water and surrounding communities. Then what? Think about smoking. A cigarette releases numerous chemicals (more than 7,000) and out of them about 70 are carcinogens as

described earlier. These harmful agents can exert cytotoxic or genotoxic effects on almost every organ in the body by damaging DNA and causing gene mutations, leading to the initiation of cancer.

2. It brings more intensified exposure to toxins as a result of rising temperature. Heat itself can make some volatile chemicals either more poisonous or unstable with unpredictable fallouts.

3. Warmer weather drives more bacterial growth. Bacteria influence cancer through provoking chronic inflammation and producing bacterial metabolites such as carcinogenic end products.

4. It brings increased diffusion of ultraviolet (UV) radiation by depleting stratospheric ozone (i.e., good ozone). As you know, the overexposure to UV radiation causes skin cancer. Noticeably, UV radiation also suppresses some aspects of immunity, thereby weakening your defense against cancer.

5. It also affects air quality by generating ground-level ozone (i.e., bad ozone) and by increasing outdoor air pollutants (especially through wildfires or storms). The IARC has classified outdoor air pollution as a human carcinogen [Group 1], and documented that ambient air pollution is a cause of lung cancer.[61] Emerging evidence indicates that extensive or long-term exposure to air pollutants has been linked to exacerbated lung diseases such as COPD and lung cancer.

6. Finally, climate change may create food safety hazards because a rise in temperature can increase natural contamination produced by fungi. One of the potential dangers is increased aflatoxin contamination of some agricultural crops or food grains. Liver cancer has been

attributed to dietary exposure to aflatoxins, a known carcinogen.[20]

Since health consequences due to climate crisis are inevitable, it is worth drawing attention to diverse factors that come with a warming climate yet may play a substantial role in cancer morbidity and mortality. We need to safeguard precious natural resources and food supply chains. Meanwhile, modify lifestyle behaviors and our exposure to outdoor air pollution. Importantly, protect sensitive individuals and vulnerable populations such as children and the elderly because they are more susceptible to weather- and air pollution-related illnesses.

Collectively, climate change can impact cancer risk, cancer development, and for sure, cancer care. Any misconception about global warming is relatively naïve and potentially dangerous.

By now, it is also clear that one critical way to prevent cancer is to reduce the exposure to environmental carcinogens.

Chapter 7 ————————————————

Radiation

A few major forms of radiation will be covered, including ultraviolet (UV) radiation, *x*-rays and *gamma* rays (ionizing radiation), and cell phones (radiofrequency radiation or nonionizing radiation).

What You Need to Know about UV Radiation

Yes, here comes the sun! And we all enjoy it. Humans live with many benefits from the sun as do many organisms, including plants, animals, and microorganisms. But did you know that more than 90 percent of skin cancer is caused by excessive exposure to the sun?

So let's face the sun's unfavorable side by examining some harmful effects of UV radiation, particularly a causal link to skin cancer.

Sunlight is the major source of UV rays, and UV radiation is a known human carcinogen. It's an unwelcome truth.

Our skin is a natural target of UV radiation. Excessive exposure to UV radiation is the most significant yet preventable risk factor for skin cancer.

Skin cancer is the most common type of cancer in fair-skinned populations in many parts of the world, including the United

States. A shocking reality is that the morbidity and mortality of skin cancers are increasing! More than 2 million Americans are diagnosed with skin cancers annually.

Melanoma is a malignant type of skin cancer. Although it accounts for only about 1 percent of skin cancers, the rate of melanoma has been rising over the last thirty years. Based on data in 2018 from the ACS, more than 91,000 people will be diagnosed with melanoma (the deadliest type of skin cancer), and about 9,320 people will die of the disease. It's also expected that during the same year, 5.4 million cases will result in the diagnosis of other less serious types of skin cancer.

Excessive exposure to the sun's UV rays is the main cause.

It's equally important to recognize some nonsolar UV exposure in our lives and in the workplace. Specifically, indoor tanning is carcinogenic to humans [Group 1] classified by the IARC.[62] Some common sources where UV is used for a variety of purposes include

- o tanning beds and sunlamps,
- o UV therapy or phototherapy,
- o black lights (referring to fluorescent lights, which are a part of UV radiation because they emit UVA rays),
- o arc welding,
- o plasma cutting torches,
- o UV nail curing lamps,
- o bacterial lamps (used in medical and dental practices for killing bacteria), and
- o high-pressure xenon and xenon-mercury arc lamps.

Who are vulnerable to a potential risk for UV damage?

Sunbathers or outdoor recreational enthusiasts are open to the risk. Outdoor or construction workers are also endangered.

Occupational workers such as dermatologists, dentists or dental assistants, laboratory staffs, welders, plasma torch operators, and salon workers are at risk as well.

Why is UV radiation harmful?

The main clinical manifestation of UV exposure can be classified into *immediate effects*, including sunburn, tanning, vitamin D production, and various skin disorders as well as deterioration because of these ailments, and *long-term effects*, including skin aging and skin cancer.

UV exposure in children under ten years old has been linked to an increased risk of developing melanoma and nonmelanoma skin cancers later in life.

Let's examine specific key factors and vital damages.

Key factors

1. The amount of UV radiation reaching the Earth's surface depends on ozone depletion, increased UV light, latitude, altitude, and weather conditions.
2. The amount of solar UV received by children and teenagers makes up 40 to 50 percent of total UV for individuals living to age sixty.
3. Unnecessary exposure to the sun and artificial UV radiation (e.g., tanning lamps) creates a personally attributable risk, and it's a significant one.
4. Hereditary or familial melanoma accounts for approximately a tenth of all melanoma cases.

Vital damages

UV radiation is a well-known carcinogen. The effects of UV radiation are primarily mediated via direct damage to DNA in the skin cells and through immune suppression.[63, 64] The severity of the effect depends on the wavelength, intensity, and duration of exposure.

- All wavelengths of UV radiation cause DNA damage to skin cells. DNA damage includes mutations, single strand breaks, inter-strand cross-links, and nucleotide base alterations. Unrepaired damages then trigger genotoxic stress and induce genome instability.
- UV-induced immune suppression contributes considerably to the growth of skin malignancies—both melanoma and nonmelanoma skin cancer. One of the immune defenses is an important surveillance system that maintains genomic integrity through cell cycle checkpoints. Once these checkpoint mechanisms sense any abnormal DNA structures, they execute cell cycle arrest and/or coordinate with the DNA repair process.
- Chronic inflammatory disorders can result from cumulative exposure to UV radiation. Other than causing skin cancers, sunburn and accelerated skin aging, UV radiation is also an environmental factor responsible for juvenile and adult myositis and other myopathies.

Adverse health effect of UV radiation is also manifested in the eyes. The eyes are very sensitive to UV rays. Damages can include flash burns, pain resulting from short exposure, watering eyes, blurred vision, and other disorders or injuries.[65]

It is important to remember that childhood is a susceptible window for long-term harmful effects of UV radiation.

Seven Signs You've Overlooked UV Radiation Damage

Sun enthusiasts, lovers of the outdoors, and many of us love doing things outside or taking a sunny beach vacation. It's a lifestyle we take for granted.

Imagine this. From overindulging in the sun, you can lose part of your ear or skin on your face, or even more serious, you can lose your life because of skin cancer. It's terrifying!

The sun is a major source of UV rays. And common skin cancers usually appear on sun-exposed areas, such as the ears, nose, and eyelids.

The sun emits three types of invisible UV rays—UVA, UVB, and UVC. It injures the human skin primarily through UVA and UVB. UVA rays are responsible for rashes and allergic reactions, while UVB rays are blamed for sunburns. Surely, both UVA and UVB speed up skin aging. However, on a more serious note, they cause skin cancer.

These harmful effects vary with seasons, time of the day, and location on the planet related to the sun. For instance, the rays are strongest between eleven in the morning and three in the afternoon in the summer. The threat of UVC rays is negligible since they are essentially blocked by the ozone layer.

Certainly, nobody wants to endure unnecessary UV treatment—by that, I mean the overexposure to UV radiation—whether it's from the sun or from tanning beds. It can undeniably increase the risk of skin cancer. Are you aware of your behaviors? Have you overlooked UV radiation damage?

While you're having fun, check out the following seven signs:

1. You may not be practicing sun protection attentively. Particularly, you didn't put on sunscreen when you went

outdoors. Nonetheless, some experts recommend applying sunscreen all year.

2. You may have had excessive or chronic exposure to the sun. I'm not suggesting that sunbathing enthusiasts should give up their pleasure. The point is that unreasonable sun exposure is costly health-wise and has proven to be hazardous to your well-being and life-threatening.

3. You may have had too much tanning. Those indoor tanning beds actually expose you to higher amounts of UV radiation.

4. Your sunscreen products may have been inadequate. Remember that all sunscreens are not created equally.

5. You may not have had a spot or mole check for some time. Be extra vigilant about any changes in spots or moles. Asking family members or a friend to help you check or visiting a dermatologist can save your life.

6. Do you lack sun-safety education? If your occupation is outdoors, but neither you nor your employer has taken sensible precautions on sun safety, then you should. Are your sunglasses UV absorbent? Have you gathered any information or knowledge on sun damage?

7. Have you been careless about the environment or ecosystem? What does this have to do with UV radiation or skin cancer? Well, a lot. Pollution and ozone layer depletion decrease our atmosphere's natural protection, which facilitates UV penetration and thus intensifies our exposure to harmful UV radiation.

Have you missed any of these signs? Now it's the time to check your sun protection measures!

SHADE—Five Essential Ways to Prevent Skin Cancer

Skin cancer remains one of most common cancers in the United States and worldwide. Fortunately, it is one of the most preventable types of cancer! Avoiding excessive sun exposure can prevent more than 90 percent of skin cancer.

Everybody loves the sun! However, you can suffer serious consequences from overexposure. Just like anything else, moderation is a key, particularly for those folks at a higher risk of skin cancer (i.e., those with recreational exposure to the sun and a history of sunburn).

Stick to the following guide that can protect you from sun damage and skin cancer. The acronym SHADE is also a handy way to remember the keys to your skin health.

S stands for "Sunscreen application."

This is an important sun-safe practice. A wide variety of sunscreens are available on the market, but not all products are created equal. It's critical to apply sunscreen with a sun protection factor (SPF) rating of 15 or higher that can block both UVA and UVB. Apply it generously to the parts of the skin that will be exposed to the sun. SPF 15 provides protection fifteen times longer before sunburn. Accordingly, SPF 30 provides protection thirty times longer.

In addition, use a moisturizer with SPF 15 or higher on a daily basis. Don't skip a day because your skin will be exposed to UV rays even on a cloudy day.

H stands for "Hide from the sun."

Skin is the largest organ in the body. It's pivotal to preserve its function. Whether you stroll under the sun or enjoy outdoors adventures, wear sunglasses and a hat, and cover up with loose clothing. Also, make sure your sunglasses have both UVA- and UVB-blocking properties.

A stands for "Avoid the sun during its most intensive time."

Staying away from the sun is especially paramount between the hours of eleven in the morning and three in the afternoon because during this window of time, the sun is at its strongest, thereby making this time the riskiest for sun damage. Keep a good practice of reasonable sun avoidance.

D stands for "Detect early, and defend daily."

Schedule an annual skin cancer screening if you are among those high-risk individuals. Also, identify early signs of skin cancer through self-awareness or attentiveness from family members and friends. Carefully examine your skin once a month, and look out for any moles, bumps, or spots that are new or changing. Notice any changes in asymmetry, border, color, diameter or size, texture, and height as well as any fluid or pain. In other words, know your ABCDEs as WebMD advised.

Sun damage is characterized by generating free radicals. Antioxidants are powerful weapons that fight or trap free radicals. So build up your antioxidant defense by eating a lot of colorful fruits and vegetables that are rich in antioxidants and micronutrients such as carotenoids, lycopene, resveratrol, and flavonoids. Eat more salmon because higher omega-3 essential fatty acids can protect you against skin damage and premature aging from UV radiation.

E stands for "Educate everyone."

Remember, E is for education, *not* entertainment under the sun! I also emphasize *everybody*. Start with children and young adults. Teach skin care equally to women and men. Regardless of gender and age, we are all exposed to the same sun.

These days the sun is getting less merciful compared to two or three decades ago because of changes in ozone protection. Thinning ozone layers in the atmosphere cannot filter out UVA and UVB radiation as effectively as they could before. Therefore, skin damage happens earlier and at a deeper level.

Let's review the five essential ways for your sun protection and skin cancer prevention.

- Sunscreen should be applied adequately.
- Hide from the sun.
- Avoid the sun during its most intensive hours.
- Detect early and defend daily.
- Educate everyone—young and old, men and women.

The acronym SHADE stands for a set of effective weapons against sun damage and skin cancer. To enjoy the great outdoors on a nice sunny day, safeguard yourself and your family by following this advice!

Medical Usage of X-Rays

Ionizing radiation (all types) including *x*-radiation is a known carcinogen.[20] Although *x*-rays, CT scans, and radiation therapy are advanced in medical use, repeated or high dosages of exposure to these procedures may carry a risk for the very disease being treated (e.g., cancer).

But relax. Cancer risk from medical imaging associated radiation is minimum. In particular, when diagnostic *x*-rays or CT scans are performed to detect any cancer at earlier, treatable stages, the potentially carcinogenic effect of radiation rarely occurs. Therefore, the benefit from the tests considerably outweighs the risk.

With that said, reduce your exposure to radiation from *x*-rays as much as possible with the following safety tips:

1. Avoid unnecessary *x*-rays.
2. When the physicians or dentists prescribe it, make sure it's absolutely necessary for a diagnostic or therapeutic purpose.
3. Use the protective shield available at the facility during a test to minimize exposure.
4. Ensure your record keeping so that any of your *x*-rays or CT scans taken previously can be transferred to prevent unnecessary exposure in the future.

Finally, as a precaution, learning the greater risk associated with pediatric radiation exposure, parents should have raised awareness to ensure the use of the least amount of radiation necessary for your children when they have to undergo medical imaging or treatment.

Cell Phone Usage and Cancer Risk Concerns

Do you use a mobile phone or cell phone? Likely, the answer is "Yes."

Advanced and popular technologies such as mobile phones have a significant impact on our communication and convenience in a fast-paced modern life. However, there may be some health concerns coming with cell phone usage.

Here, I'll draw your attention to a couple of important matters regarding cell phone safety because of its radiation concern, and help you understand why and how to protect yourself from potential cancer risk and health hazards without compromising your convenience.

Where does cell phone radiation go?

Cell phones work by emitting radiofrequency (RF) radiation (i.e., nonionizing radiation), which is different from UV and x-rays (ionizing radiation). Cell phone radiation is weaker than UV rays and x-rays but stronger than FM radio signal. Cell phone radiation strength is measured by specific absorption rate (SAR).

A part of the RF waves given off by cell phones is absorbed by the human head or body, and the other parts can go into air (i.e., environment). So it's considerate if one tries not to passively expose others to the phone's RF electromagnetic fields, especially in crowded public settings.

Does cell phone usage cause cancer?

First, there is a possible link between cell phone use and cancer risk, especially brain tumor development. Research shows that cell phone usage is associated with an increased risk of some cancers in humans, mainly brain tumors such as glioma (a malignant brain tumor) and other cancer of the central nervous system. Swedish researchers found a close association between the long-term usage of cell phones and increased risk of brain tumor.[66] Studies also confirm that the frequent or heavy mobile phone users are likely to develop tumors on the same side of their brain that they put to use their devices. Regardless of a few controversies, the IARC has classified radiofrequency electromagnetic fields as possibly carcinogenic to humans.[67] This implies personal exposure through mobile phone usage.

Second, children are more vulnerable to the potential carcinogenic effects of mobile radiation exposure. Their vulnerability may be based on (1) the thinner skull for RF radiation's penetration, (2) a smaller head size for relatively greater RF penetration, (3) a greater sensitivity of their developing nervous systems, and (4) their longer lifetime of exposure. Notably, a child's brain absorbs up to twice as much RF as an adult's brain.[68]

Finally, cumulative exposure to mobile radiation may be attributed to various factors. Consider the number of cell phone calls per day, the length of each call, and the amount of time (including years) using a cell phone. Keep in mind that the RF dose intensity depends on the distance between the device and the body because mobile phones emit RF radiation constantly through communicating with cell towers.

Taken together, it is wise to take precautions. Moreover, cell phone usage does cause some health problems related to the location of the body, time or magnitude of exposure, such as damaged sperms and skin illnesses.

What are the best strategies for cell phone users to protect yourself and your family from cancer risk?

1. Use moderately (or limit its use).
2. Use when the signal is good and strong.
3. Keep it away from your head if possible, or use the speakerphone function.
4. Make conversations short.
5. Turn it off whenever it's not in use.
6. Use a cell phone with the lowest SAR possible.
7. Allow minimal usage for children. The cell phone is not a toy for kids but a tool. It's a long-term protection for kids if they only use when absolutely necessary or in the case of emergencies.
8. Don't sleep with your cell phone. Keep it out of your bedroom to optimize your sleep.

Deposit old or used cell phones conscientiously. Some components of cell phones such as antennas, speakers, and keypads are small in size but contain heavy metals and hazardous materials, which is not environmentally friendly.

Keys to Being Mobile Friendly While Staying Protected Wisely

Mobile technology has not just grown popular. It has become a necessity. Mobile phone uses expand far beyond keeping connections with families and friends and conducting business. Today you can enjoy conveniences ranging from information about thousands of topics, entertainment, self-learning to mobile banking, mobile wallet, and innovative health care.

But as convenient and useful as they are, smartphones also invite some serious consequences, including cancer risk from radiation, especially for brain tumors and other health hazards (e.g., male infertility, neurological disorders, metabolic syndromes and sleep troubles). The most immediate life-threatening danger is from traffic accidents, which may occur while someone is driving and messaging or conversing on the phone simultaneously. Lighter problems may include pains in the fingers, tendons, neck, or back that otherwise are without a clear explanation.

So how do you become mobile friendly while maintaining wellness wisely?

Here are some thought-provoking questions to evaluate your well-being and protect your treasure (i.e., your health):

- Is there another way available to obtain your desired results with little or no radiation? If so, take the alternative way.
- Is a poor signal a warning sign against radiation harm? If so, stop or shorten the conversation.

- Before purchasing a new cell phone, ask or search for answers to questions about radiation output. Does this device emit the most intensive radiation? Make sure your tech source is reliable.
- On the road, could the conversation you are in potentially destroy you? Using hands-free headsets are not accident-proof!
- Are privacy and data safety of concern to you? If so, get rid of this stressor.
- Gentlemen, do you keep your cell phones away from your pants whenever possible?
- Are you aware of your posture when you are focused on your mobile devices? A poor posture is a red flag for various health issues.
- Are you conscious about passive radiation that may affect others, especially in a crowded public setting? Remember that nonionizing radiation from cell phones goes not only to the human brain but also to the air!
- Do you dispose of your cell phones in an eco-friendly way?

Three pointers for protecting your kids

1. Intentionally postpone early childhood exposure, and tactically limit your children's mobile use because they face a longer lifetime exposure to any hidden health hazards.
2. Clean your children's cell phones often, and train them to practice this habit daily because a cell phone is a safe haven for many bacteria, including antibiotic-resistant superbugs.
3. As a rule of thumb, say no to mobile devices during bedtime. Be the angel and protector of your children!

Chapter 8

Infection

Infection Is a Risk Factor for Cancer

Infections are everywhere and occur in many types, including flu, food poisoning, tick-borne Lyme disease, and many other forms (e.g., meningitis and hepatitis). The consequences of infections vary anywhere from a temporary sickness or harmful condition to long-term diseases.

Infectious agents (e.g., bacteria and viruses) can cause cancer too. Here I'd like to highlight the role of infection in cancer development and to some extent, in chronic illnesses.

Role of bacteria in cancer

There is a significant association between infection and a risk of cancer.[69] For example, the following bacteria or microbial pathogens are responsible for an increased risk of certain cancers:

- *Helicobacter pylori* (H. pylori), a known carcinogen, is linked to stomach cancer and lymphoma.
- *Salmonella typhi* infection is linked to gallbladder cancer.[70]
- *Chlamydia pneumoniae* is linked to lung cancer.

- *Chlamydia* infection is linked to ovarian cancer and cervical cancer.
- *Neisseria gonorrhoeae* is linked to cancers of the bladder, ovaries, and prostate.
- *Schistosoma* is linked to bladder cancer.[71, 72]

The microbial community in the human colon is gigantic. Emerging data imply an association between multiple bacterial species with colorectal cancer development. Some of the bacteria responsible for the multiphase process include *Bacteroides fragilis, Streptococcus gallolyticus, Fusobacterium* species, *Salmonella* species, and *Escherichia coli.*[73-75]

Specifically, Bacteroides fragilis and Escherichia coli are involved in developing colon cancer, especially among people with familial adenomatous polyposis (FAP), an inherited disorder in which multiple benign polyps grow in the colon with a high risk of turning malignant. This is because the two strains can bypass the gut barrier that acts as an intestinal guardian, and reach the epithelial cells (i.e., cells that line the insides of organs, including the gastrointestinal tract), turning these cells cancerous.

Although research has shown that certain bacteria are associated with human cancers, their role in cancer is complex. Compelling evidence links some species to the growth of cancer while others appear promising in the diagnosis, prevention, or treatment of cancers. However, you might wonder how bacterial infection could lead to cancer.

Bacteria may cause cancer through the following:

- **Chronic infection**

Some bacterial toxins can negatively impact the process that controls normal cell cycle and cell growth. Others disrupt the cellular signaling pathways that regulate normal cell death, consequently promoting cancer development. In addition, infection-induced immune response may release immune modulating substances from inflammatory cells, contributing to carcinogenesis.

- **DNA damage**

Bacteria can produce free radicals, which are very unstable and highly reactive with other molecules. Bacteria also release toxins that are genotoxic. These bacterial products can bind to DNA and cause DNA mutation, thereby altering the genes that control normal cell division and cell death. Accumulated mutations drive increased proliferation, leading to malignancies. Cancer is initiated when uncontrolled growth of abnormal cells takes place.

- **Weakened or suppressed immune system**

The immune system is a central line of defense against any toxins or diseases, including cancer. Toxins or pathogens sometimes can get away from the host's immune system to survive and then modify one's immune function. When its function is compromised, the immune system no longer recognizes and fights bacteria or toxins as foreign bodies. Nor does it get rid of them.

That being said, don't panic. A majority of individuals will not develop cancer after infection by a cancer-causing agent. However, be conscious and alert. The facts are as follows:

1. Certain individuals are more susceptible to cancer-causing infections.
2. Incidents of certain cancers may vary among populations or geographic regions.
3. It often takes years or decades between acquiring the infection and getting cancer.

Role of viruses in cancer

A growing body of knowledge indicates that viruses can cause cancer.[20, 76] Here are some well-documented cases:

-   Hepatitis B virus is a proven cause of liver cancer.
-   Hepatitis C virus contributes to liver cancer and non-Hodgkin lymphoma.
-   Human immunodeficiency virus (HIV) participates in anal and cervical cancer, Kaposi sarcoma, Hodgkin lymphoma, and non-Hodgkin lymphoma.
-   Human papillomavirus (HPV) is an established cause of cervical cancer, and contributes to cancers of the mouth, pharynx, anus, vulva, vagina, ovary, penis, and lungs (likely in non-smokers).
-   Human herpes virus type-8 (Kaposi sarcoma herpes virus, KSHV) is a cause of Kaposi sarcoma and lymphoma.
-   Epstein bar virus (EBV) is a known carcinogen evident in lymphoma, Hodgkin lymphoma, gastric and nasopharyngeal cancer.

Cancers occur when the genetic material (i.e., DNA) within the cells develops mutations that lead to uncontrolled cell growth. The mutations may result from damage in DNA structure or errors in DNA replication.

Like bacteria, viruses can play a role in tumorgenesis through direct or indirect mechanisms. Distinctively, viruses can insert themselves into the cell's DNA, causing the same mutation and consequence, i.e., genomic instability. Also, viruses can trigger chronic inflammation, produce secondary tissue damage, and cause immunosuppression, thereby favoring the development of cancer in host cells.

An estimated 12 to 20 percent of human cancers are caused

by viruses. Because there is no vaccine available for some viruses, prevention is critical to protect you from cancer risks.

Keep in mind that impacts from bacteria, viruses, and other pathogens on our health not only manifest in infectious diseases but also play a lasting role in certain cancers or other chronic illnesses.

Why infection should not be overlooked

The infection may be gone, but the risk may not. And the infection may be going on, but the symptoms may not show.

As mentioned above, it's scientifically and clinically proven that infection is a risk factor of cancer. Consider that H. pylori (a bacterium responsible for gastritis, gastric ulcer and cancer) infects the gastric ecosystem in 50 percent of all humans. Once H. pylori settles in the gastric environment, it stays for the lifetime of a host.

Pancreatic inflammation may increase the risk of pancreatic cancer. It's been shown that some patients with pancreatic cancer had a history of pancreatitis. A history of urinary tract infection is accepted as a risk factor for developing bladder cancer and renal cell carcinoma (kidney cancer). Men with a history of smoking have a notably elevated risk for these diseases.

Some of common cancers are attributed to infectious agents yet asymptomatic. HPV (also called the wart virus) is responsible for cervical cancer, one of the most common cancers affecting women. A twofold danger exists with this disease. First, HPV is highly transmissible and considered the most common sexually transmissible infection in most populations. Second, most women infected with the virus may appear negative in the test within two years, and HPV infection can persist for years in the body without causing any problems. In the end, women with persistent

HPV infections are at the greatest risk for developing cervical cancer.

My father had pulmonary tuberculosis nearly four decades ago. Clinically, it had been thought as healed tuberculosis after timely treatment along with years of monitoring. Even until two years before the diagnosis of lung cancer, the only thing showing on his chest x-ray was a localized calcification (i.e., calcium deposition, a mark of healed lesion in his case) without any visible changes. Also, he was symptomless when it came to any upper-respiratory diseases. Unexpectedly, there was lung malignancy clearly showing on his last chest x-ray—one that appeared significantly different compared with the one taken two years prior.

Countless similar stories tell of the connection between personal histories of infectious diseases and cancer. A friend of mine died of liver cancer in his 40s. The tragedy came shockingly fast and vicious. It turned out that he had hepatitis (infected with hepatitis B virus) when he was young.

We can go on and on. It's dangerous to ignore infections.

This doesn't mean that you'll develop cancer if you have any infection or inflammation. Infection alone usually does not lead to cancer. However, it does mean that you need to control your infection, get it treated in a timely manner, be vigilant about any cancer risk factors, and live a healthy lifestyle.

Overall, it's evident that a variety of infectious agents are linked to numerous chronic diseases. Infection and subsequent chronic inflammation can increase the risk of cancer. Therefore, it is crucial to eliminate the cause of infection when it arises by getting timely treatment. The best measure you can take before infection occurs is to prevent infection in the first place.

And that is why I want to emphasize the danger of infections and the value of prevention.

Prevention is key

Here are some effective strategies and tips for prevention.

1. *Be hygiene-conscious.* Wash your hands. This is a very important health practice. Sounds simple, right? However, not everybody does it. Let me elaborate a bit more because good hand-washing is very effective for blocking a contact-oral or fecal-oral route of infection.

    First, wash your hands frequently, especially after using the bathroom, handling trash, or touching any dirty surfaces and before eating food. Wash thoroughly with soap over the entirety of the hands, not just a quick rinse of the palms.

    Next, I always recommend people to wash your hands after touching cash. The concern with cash is not how many people have touched it but who have handled it. It's a huge unknown that makes cash potentially contagious.

    Equally important is to teach kids to do this too. It takes time to develop habits. Cultivating this heathy habit provides them with considerable lifelong protection.

2. *Maintain food hygiene.* One way that germs enter a human body is through the mouth. So carefully watch what you eat and drink. For example, wash fruits and vegetables before eating them, and cook meats, fish, and seafood fully. It's also better not to share utensils.

    The intake of contaminated food or water can result in salmonella infection or becoming infected with other pathogens such as hepatitis virus. And it takes at least boiling in water at 100 degrees Celsius (212 degrees Fahrenheit) to kill the hepatitis virus. That's why chewing ice cubes is not always cool unless you know the exact water source of the ice.

3. *Become vigilant about the hygiene of your surrounding area.* This includes keeping clean the kitchen area where foods are prepared and preventing hospital-associated infections. When traveling, be aware of common surfaces with germs, such as door handles and keypads used for many cashless tasks or transactions.

4. *Practice sex hygiene.* Sexually transmitted infections can lead to cancer and death, and not all of them can be cured. Get immunized, get to know your partner, avoid reckless sexual behavior, and apply safe measures to reduce the risk of infections.

5. *Get vaccinated.* Vaccines represent a highly effective anticancer strategy. Vaccination is vital because it helps protect not only you but also the people around you and your communities.

6. *Support your immune function and minimize inflammation.* Your immune system is the front line of your body's defense against toxins and diseases, including cancer. (See more solutions and tips for effective immune-boosting in the book.)

In brief, practicing good hygiene and developing habits that foster strong immunity are beneficial for your long-term health.

Twenty-Five Unbeatable Ways to Strengthen Your Immune System

Your immune system is your body's natural defense against diseases. Its functions range from fighting off harmful bacteria and viruses to destroying potentially cancerous cells.

However, our immune systems are under attack in our daily lives from a variety of sources—free radicals, bacteria, UV radiation, environmental pollutants, and stress. It's critical not only to ensure your immune system is always healthy but to maximize its functional capacity as well. Luckily, there are actions we can take to achieve this goal.

1. Eat a healthy diet. Mindfully include immune-boosting foods in everyday meals.
2. Exercise and be physically active. You can do all-body workouts, running, walking, and dancing, and/or gardening. The key is to keep moving.
3. Cultivate a new hobby that's physically demanding, makes your heart beat faster and your blood circulate better. As a result, you'll become more fit.
4. Practice quietness. Enjoy tranquility. A quiet mind may promote inner peace and relaxation.
5. Take a hot bath or shower. Soaking in a warm bath is another way of relaxing.
6. Get enough sleep. Lack of sleep or sleep deprivation can impair your immune functions.
7. Reduce stress. Everybody gets stress from different areas of life. There's a long list of stress management tips, but not all work for everyone. Have fun discovering and developing whatever works for you.

8. Be kind. According to a good friend of mine who is an experienced oncologist, my dad's prolonged life was certainly attributed to his extraordinary kindness.

9. Appreciate the little things in life, and always maintain a positive and grateful attitude. Research suggests that individuals with a negative frame of mind have more difficulty properly maintaining their immune response and thereby pose a higher risk for illness compared to those with a positive attitude.

10. Get outdoors. Whether you walk, ski, bike, or hike, the combination of enjoying the beauty of nature and a dose of exercise boosts your immune system.

11. Maintain a clutter-free home and workplace because clutter is a stress trigger. Clear those mental clutters too.

12. Laugh and smile often. Laughter boosts your immune system at no cost. The more folks laugh, the less depression they experience. If you have any difficulty laughing, go for "laughter yoga" by checking out a local group that practices it.

13. Have a sense of humor. Yes, some people have more of a funny bone than others. Yet many people just don't foster their funny side, a dimension that almost everyone possesses in some ways.

14. Practice deep breathing to stay calm. Count to three before any anger takes over.

15. Nurture your emotional well-being. Be happy. If you don't promote emotional health, your physical body will pay the price. Emotions are intimately involved in the initiation and progression of cancer, cardiovascular disease, and HIV.

16. Take time off, and take breaks during the day.

17. Eat a healthy breakfast, not just any breakfast. Skipping breakfast is even worse.
18. Maintain a healthy weight. Remember that it could be a fun marathon rather than an overnight remedy.
19. Stop eating sugar. Sugar suppresses the immune system. Even a teaspoon of sugar can reduce the activity of your body's natural killer cells for hours. There are many wonderful foods that help improve your immune function. Explore them to replace sugar.
20. Eat more soups, especially chicken soup.
21. Drink a lot of water. If possible, filter your drinking/cooking water.
22. Drink more tea, especially green tea.
23. Get plenty of fresh air. In particular, keep your indoor air clean and fresh.
24. Deal with any health concern, even pain or an unusual spot as soon as possible. Fix any small problem for the optimal function of the big machine, namely your body.
25. Develop good relationships around you. A strong family bond, a happy marriage, and good friendships can help you during good and tough times.

Nutritious food is the best and natural immune-booster. If you have to take multivitamin or mineral supplements to ensure an adequate supply of the essential nutrients that are needed by your body yet lacking from your diet, make sure to take a quality-controlled supplement rather than just any supplement as the dietary supplements are virtually unregulated. Consult with your physician too.

Our immune system is effective most of the time. Following the above tips will remarkably boost your immune system and promote your happiness.

Twenty Don'ts to Improve Your Immunity and Lower Cancer Risk

While eating a balanced diet is essential, healthy eating habits are equally important for the immune system. Why? Because poor eating manners or habits cause poor digestion, which can result in poor nutrition by affecting nutrient breakdown, absorption, and metabolism, and can leave toxins to accumulate in the body, thereby leading to an overstressed immune system.

Accordingly, what are the habits that could be harmful to your immune system? Follow this list to get rid of them.

1. Don't eat too much for each meal. A golden rule is— Control your food intake to 70 to 80 percent full, and fill the rest with two to three snacks throughout the day.
2. Don't overeat at once. The worst is bringing an empty stomach to a party or buffet and eating a huge meal. Overeating is one of the triggers for illnesses.
3. Don't skip meals for whatever reasons. Don't ever skip your breakfast. Eating no food cannot make you slim.
4. Don't ingest too much sugar (e.g., eating sugar-rich deserts or drinking sweetened beverages).
5. Don't eat too much salty food. High sodium contributes to hypertension and cardiovascular diseases.
6. Don't eat too much food that's high in fat, especially animal fats, saturated and trans fats.
7. Don't eat very hot food. Asian folks are accustomed to having warm dishes, but some of them tend to eat a dish when it's still quite hot. Hot food hurts the esophagus.
8. Don't eat very spicy food. It can injure the cells of the esophagus and stomach, subsequently causing poor digestion and weakening the immune system.

9. Don't eat a meat-oriented diet, especially red meat and processed meat.

10. Don't eat too many animal organs. For instance, the liver is an abundant source for protein, vitamins, and minerals as well as the largest organ for detoxification. Because toxins are mostly processed and excreted through the liver, many toxins are also hidden there.

11. Don't eat processed foods as your daily diet. Processed foods contain more fats, salts, sugar and possibly known carcinogens but lack the vital nutrients necessary to support immune functions.

12. Don't dislike food. Eat a diversity of foods to get those nutrients that are not contained in one food and to avoid nutrient imbalance. If you really *hate* a particular one, always substitute it with another from the same family with similar nutrients.

13. Don't eat too many fast foods.

14. Don't eat too fast. Enjoy your meal!

15. Don't eat too much before going to bed. It's amazing how many people eat a big dinner before bedtime.

16. Don't eat or take something blindly. In other words, don't go with the marketing flow. For example, ginseng's effects on the body could be good or excellent, but is not good for everyone.

17. Don't go without water. Drink at least eight glasses a day.

18. Don't drink alcohol excessively. Excessive alcohol damages various organs and immune functions.

19. Don't drink too many soft drinks or artificial juices.

20. Don't forget to maintain food hygiene. Dirt on fruits or veggies, grease, or traces of food in the microwave provide nutrition to bacteria and invite some illnesses. Poor food hygiene affects food safety.

In short, healthy eating habits promote a strong immune system and minimize your risks for illnesses including cancer. Healthy eating takes discipline too.

Role of Inflammation in Chronic Diseases

Chronic Inflammation: A Common Root for Cancer and Cardiovascular Diseases

Do you know that the effect of inflammation can be twofold?

Inflammation is a reaction to bacterial or viral infection. Under physiological conditions, injuries or infections can trigger natural, healthy immune responses, and acute inflammation is an important part of the healing process.

However, when the immune-stimulated inflammation persists, it becomes a toxic driver of chronic illnesses, causing cells in vital organs to dysfunction or degenerate.

Chronic inflammation has been linked to a variety of health problems such as cancer, heart disease, diabetes, depression, and Alzheimer's disease.[77, 78]

How can inflammation lead to deadly diseases?

1. Chronic inflammation caused by a variety of infectious agents can promote development of cancer by the release of immune modulating factors/substances, the production of DNA-damaging free radicals, and the suppression of immune functions.

2. Sufficient evidence shows that chronic inflammation in fat tissue plays a key role in insulin resistance, e.g., inflammation-promoting cytokines make the body less

sensitive to insulin, leading to elevated levels of blood sugar and then type 2 diabetes.

3. Obesity is considered a chronic inflammatory disease. Furthermore, abdominal obesity is a risk factor for various diseases linked to inflammation. Fat cells around the belly are much more biologically active than those under the skin, and they release some hormones and inflammatory chemicals. Obesity has been linked to several types of cancer.[79, 80]

4. Fat and cholesterol surely build up plaque on the arterial walls. Additionally, undetected chronic infection or inflammation participates in the formation of vulnerable plaque, which means that an unstable clot can easily fall off the arterial wall and travel to the heart or brain, resulting in myocardial infarction or stroke.

What can trigger inflammation?

1. **Poor diet**: Baseline nutrition is critical, at least, to maintain necessary levels of anti-inflammatory nutrients in the body. Heavy alcohol consumption can lead to chronic inflammation.

2. **High-fat, high-sugar, and high-salt foods**: They're tasty, but they are silent fuels that can set your body on fire.

3. **Toxic chemicals**: Environmental pollutants (from tobacco to asbestos to dangerous chemicals in our home or workplace) that in the air we breathe and water we drink can be inflammatory sources.

4. **Stress**: Emotional or mental and physical stress can make the immune system overdrive and cause an imbalance

between inflammatory and anti-inflammatory responses followed by chronic inflammation.

5. **Physical inactivity**: Sedentary behaviors upregulate inflammatory signaling pathways. Exercise can produce beneficial changes in the circulating insulin or insulin-related pathways and in eliminating inflammatory mediators.

The significant role that chronic inflammation plays in some killer diseases is clear, and the information here can empower you to control chronic inflammation in various ways.

Chapter 9 ——————————

Aging and Uncontrollable Factors

Age Is a Primary Risk Factor for Cancer

Age itself is uncontrollable, but aging as a process, though inevitable, is controllable. Healthy aging is about living well, not just living long.

Aging cells and cancer cells are opposite. Aging cells are senescence (i.e., elderliness) and die. In contrast, cancer cells are eternal because they can grow and divide indefinitely.

A blossoming body of knowledge has presented us with various factors that accelerate or slow down aging. There are proven, personal, and expanded approaches to aging, which I'm excited to share with you.

So let's dive in.

How do you define aging?

Aging is characterized by a structural and functional degradation or adaptation, variably affecting multiple body systems because of a complex interaction among genetic, environmental, and random factors.

Simply speaking, aging is a complex process through a progressive loss of physical integrity, which has a negative impact on various body systems and a deteriorated effect on biological functions.

As we age, our bodies go through a lot of changes. My focus is on those changes associated with some vital organs and cancer development.

Why age is a primary risk factor for cancer

An older age is the greatest risk factor for developing cancer. According to statistical data, more than half of all cancers occur in people age 66 or older.

Why cancer risk increases as you age is not completely clear. There is no single explanation for why an aging body is more susceptible to cancer. However, here are a few possibilities:[81-83]

Firstly, because cancer doesn't strike overnight, one explanation could be that DNA damage—the root of developing cancerous cells and a multifaceted process—takes place over a long period of time through intrinsic and extrinsic factors. Inside the body ROS from cellular metabolism cause DNA damage and mutation, and so do prolonged, accumulated exposures to carcinogens from external sources, such as sun/UV radiation, bacteria or viruses, and environmental toxins or pollutants in the air, the water, and the food. (See the illustration on how DNA damage contributes to aging and cancer.)

Flowchart Illustration 3. How DNA damage contributes to aging and cancer

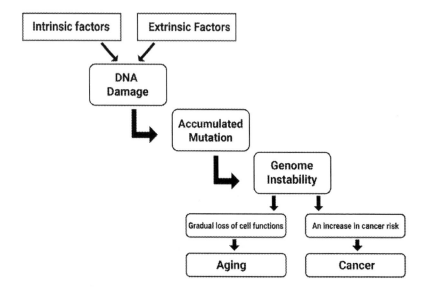

Secondly, a human's immunity is the frontline defense against cancer. However, our immune system tends to decline or get weaker over the course of our lifetimes. As you age, collected damages to the cells put an increased burden on your immune response. The weakened immune system is less vigilant in detecting cancerous cells, less effective in attacking them, and less resilient in fighting infections and diseases.

Thirdly, we must think about telomeres. Telomeres are like caps on chromosomes with repetitive DNA sequences, and most telomeres shrink after each cell division. Thus biologically, telomere length shortens as we age. Unlike other genomic elements, telomeres are very sensitive to stress-induced DNA damage. Moreover, it's difficult to repair the damage to telomeres. When telomeres are much injured or much faded, cellular senescence takes place, which is evident with aging.[84] In the short term, however, it lowers cancer risk by closing down cellular pathways to abnormal growth or proliferation. Eventually, telomeres damage and shortening also lead to genetic instability seen in both aging and carcinogenesis,

Lastly, consider inflammation. One of the hallmarks of aging is a chronic and systematic low-grade inflammatory process. Likewise, chronic inflammation is a hallmark of cancer. Age-related alterations in cellular homeostatic apparatuses also render the aged vasculature more susceptible to the damaging effects of oxidative stress, endothelial dysfunction and chronically elevated inflammatory substances, which then accelerate vascular aging and age-related multidimensional conditions such as cancer and cardiovascular disease.[83, 85] So the aging process is biologically coupled with cancer development.

Definitely, aging and cancer share some hallmarks and risk factors (see the following table).

However, the fundamental difference is apparent. Aged cells are senescent (i.e., they are in dormant or sleep mode). Cancer cells, on the other hand, are proliferating and immortal (i.e., they are in growth or hyperactive mode).

Table 1. Similarities and differences between aging and cancer

Characteristics / Factors	Aging	Cancer
Genomic instability	Accelerated	Accelerated
Telomere shortening	Evident	Evident
Cells	Cellular senescence	Cellular growth, immortalization
Immune system	Declining, weakened	Evading or weakened
Nutrient, Metabolism	Decreased, dysregulated	Sensed & adopted alterations
Risk Factors to accelerate both processes		
Radiation	Yes	Yes
Smoking	Yes	Yes
Unhealthy diet/foods	Yes	Yes
Sedentary lifestyle	Yes	Yes
Environment toxins	Yes	Yes
Obesity	Yes	Yes
Inflammation	Yes	Yes

In a parallel way, *cancer is a disease of aging*. Age is simply a number, but aging is a process. Cancer is multifaceted and each one varies; however, all cancers develop over time.

Hopefully, we can prevent cancer by slowing down aging.

Indeed, how well we age depends on many factors, including what we eat or drink, how physically active we are, and how often and how long we are exposed to health hazards such as tobacco smoking, excessive alcohol consumption, sun or radiation, chemical toxins, etc.

Chronically stimulated inflammation together with genetic, lifestyle, and environmental risk factors can speed up the process of physiological deterioration and ailing conditions that lead to death.

After all, age drives diseases. Age is a major risk factor for the leading causes of death. The risk of death from predominant killer diseases—such as cancer, heart disease, stroke, diabetes, COPD and

Alzheimer's disease—increases dramatically with age, especially in the population living a sedentary lifestyle and eating a Western diet.

The good news is that cancer and other age-related chronic diseases are mostly preventable! Prevention can be successful through lifestyle modification or intervention.

Before I show you proven approaches to prevention, let me address how traditional Chinese medicine views successful aging and healthy lifespan.

Traditional Chinese Medicine on Aging, Illness, and Longevity

Traditional Chinese medicine (TCM) emphasizes human vitality. That implies that longevity is not about mere length of life. It is also about quality of life. That means living a life without suffering pain, distress, and diseases.

One of the fundamental principles of TCM is *qi* (pronounced *chee*), which is a life force or vital energy that flows through the body. Qi is crucial to longevity. Qi performs multiple functions in maintaining health.

In particular, this concept has no counterpart or equivalent in Western medicine.

Qi properly circulates through the body in channels or pathways (referred to *meridians*). Qi also interconnects across organs and tissues through circulating hormones, signaling molecules, nerve transmission, electrical stimuli, or environmental cues, assuring many aspects of health. Any stagnated, blocked, disrupted, or unbalanced qi can result in illnesses or symptoms. Similarly, injury, physical suffering, and poor nutrition cause qi deficiency.

For example, the root of cancer is associated with qi. One belief in TCM states that "*Flow of qi makes blood circulate; stagnation of qi causes blood stasis.*" The mass and abnormal growth of cancer essentially result from elements such as qi stagnation, blood stasis/stillness, and phlegm buildup. Remarkably, these changes are attributed to various factors, including inadequate diet, lack of exercise, emotional stress, and external pathogens or toxins.

Qi can be replenished, drained, or diminished. To sustain life, we replenish our vital energy by supporting, nurturing or building up qi, which can be achieved by the foods we ingest, the water we drink, the air we breathe, exercise, meditation, and probably more important, our emotional states and mind sets. These all influence health and healing. Simply put, everything counts as energy at physical, mental, and spiritual levels.

That's why TCM practices mainly target at unblocking qi and/or facilitating qi to flow inside the body properly. Qi gong is an exercise that helps with balancing qi through coordinated movement, rhythmic breathing, awareness, and meditative state, and it has an effect on healing.

So well-moving and intra-connected qi promotes blood circulation, regulates metabolism, and reduces inflammation, leading to optimal health.

Strategies and Secrets to Healthy Aging and Healthspan

When I take a note on the oldest old—an exceptional group of individuals with healthy longevity beyond the average life span—in documents and in real life, they are heterogeneous physiologically, socially, and demographically. And you can join the club too.

Just glancing at the gray or silver population, you can see a person of age sixty as fragile and ailing. Then you can consider Ruth Bader Ginsburg, a U.S. Supreme Court justice. At the age of eighty-six, she is an admirable example of energy, resilience, intellect, and a sharp mind. Other elderly people like my late father-in-law (at the age of ninety-three), live independent and active lives. Of course, you have many folks somewhere in between these two extremes.

Thankfully, aforementioned TCM viewpoints on longevity parallel a new concept of extending the period of life spent free from chronic disease and disability, referred to as healthspan. Many scientists aspire to explore cutting-edge research and develop new therapies targeted at extending healthspan.[86]

I have collected some key strategies and secrets for your healthspan, not just lifespan.

Ten key strategies that protect your vital qi and prevent cancer

1. **Love your age and steer clear of self-stereotype. Laugh more!**

   Your mind-set propels your feelings or actions, so maintain a positive outlook. Growing older, you are subject to grumpiness or illness just like anybody else, including youngsters. Moreover, nobody's case is as unique and exceptional as yours. Even in a broad sense, an aging body's functions decline, but the exact dynamic and pattern of changes vary from individual to individual, depending on genetic and environmental conditions. So focus on the amazing and amusing side of your life journey!

2. **Monitor your physical and emotional wellness by knowing your NICE.**

   Number is your critical numbers (blood pressure, blood sugar, cholesterol, and etc.)

In circle refers to keeping a circle of loved ones, a network of friends for care and support.

Cancer screening is self-explanatory. Consider the colon as a window into the aging gut or digestive system. Check your lung, breast or prostate regularly.

Emotion encompasses your feelings—stressful, grateful, joyful, sad, angry, or lonely on a daily basis.

Again, your body is entirely connected. So schedule routine doctor visits and cancer testing for early detection.

3. **Maintain a healthy weight and ward off abdominal obesity.**

It can be difficult with age—whether you're struggling with weight loss or just holding the line at your current weight—because of hormonal and other internal changes. The key is setting a realistic goal and making small changes daily. Excessive calorie intake and a sedentary lifestyle can cause abdominal obesity.

4. **Have a diet rich in nutrients and fibers along with sufficient water intake.**

Eat a plenty of fruits, vegetables, fish, beans, whole grains, nuts, and seeds, which are great sources of proteins, vitamins, minerals, and fibers. Ingest necessary healthy fats. Avoid or limit foods high in animal fat, sugar, and salt. To promote longevity, choose what you eat and drink wisely.

5. **Engage in physical activities daily and make it a priority.**

   Get moving, and keep going. There are many ways, small or big, to get active every day. Make sure to improve your strength, balance, and flexibility, and better yet, have fun while you do so! In the end, you gain a lot of benefits in practically every area of your later life.

6. **Quit smoking (because it's never too late to boost longevity), and foster healthy habits/behaviors.**

   Care for your oral health by brushing and flossing, and visit your dentist regularly. Keep up on your personal hygiene, food hygiene, and diet hygiene (no overeating or ingesting a big meal before bedtime).

7. **Remember to get a good night's sleep.**

   Naturally, older adults already experience a decrease in their amount of deep sleep and an increase in wakefulness during the night. Find ways to get sufficient sleep. (See more in the chapter on sleep)

8. **Practice gratitude. Gratitude is a secret to happiness.**

   Keep counting your blessings. A person once said, "There's always a lot to be thankful for if you take time to look for it. For example, I am sitting here and thinking about how nice it is that wrinkles don't hurt." That person is so content and humorous. I love it! Studies demonstrate that people who are always grateful and practice gratitude in their lives tend to have more peaceful and harmonious existences than those who do not.

9. **Love more, learn more, and live fully.**

Infuse love, interests, joy and resilience to enrich your life. Besides the love to your family and friends, you can entertain a diverse array of acts out of love, such as pursuing your passion, embracing or giving to your community, volunteering to a great cause, and reaching out to help others. Learning keeps you mentally sharp and spiritually young. Try to learn something every day and every year, whether it is from reading or from doing, whether it's a skill, art or sport. Purposefully challenge your mental ability in fun ways (e.g., puzzles, games, or writing club). Seek new experiences or new relationships.

10. **Prevent or slow down vascular aging.**

English physician Thomas Sydenham once famously said "A man is as old as his arteries." Vascular aging is accelerated by circumstances such as oxidative stress, endothelial dysfunction and chronic inflammation. With aging, the blood vessels undergo predictable changes in arterial structure and function (e.g., arterial stiffness), and become more susceptible to vascular diseases. Thus, it's critical to take care of your vasculature. The strategies and secrets described herein can also go a long way to protect your vascular integrity and help control your blood pressure. Remember that qi and blood are intimately dependent, so keep them flow freely.

If you desire to age gracefully and brilliantly, place a strong focus on these areas. Let's face it. You cannot help age or aging, but you don't have to get old. In life, we have choices. You can be a grumpy, depressed, or ailing senior or somebody healthful in body and ageless in spirit.

In the end, we all hope to achieve one of humanity's greatest dreams, which is to have a long, productive, and happy life in a healthy body.

So embrace aging. Don't just endure it. Let that ray of happiness or wholeness penetrate the cloud of gloom in the coming phase of your life.

Uncontrollable Risk Factors for Cancer

Besides age, other risk factors for cancer are basically not controllable. However, knowing each of them is still necessary in determining your overall risk and taking preventative measures. These factors are:

o   Genetic or inherited mutation
o   Family history
o   Gender
o   Race and Ethnicity
o   Previous history of cancer

Just as genes determine the color of eyes or hairs, they can directly or indirectly predispose any offspring to cancer. A person can inherit a predisposition for a certain type of cancer that in time results in malignancy, whereas another individual has a genetic susceptibility to the disease that is later triggered by an environmental or lifestyle factor.

That's why genetic screening can be beneficial, especially for people who have the disease in their family trees—first-degree relatives (parent or sibling), second-degree relatives (grandparent, grandchild, aunt or uncle), and others.

Nobody has control over their genes, family history of cancer, race or ethnicity, and gender. However, each of us can control those modifiable risk factors, choices of lifestyle, and early detection for cancer.

Early detection is one of the key strategies to prevent cancer

In addition to knowing your risk factors and genetic testing, early detection involves guided cancer screening and consultation with your physician whenever you are in doubt.

Warning signs and symptoms of cancer include

- people age fifty or older;
- any new or unusual change in the body (e.g., a lump, ulcer, or pain) that doesn't go away;
- any unexplained bleeding (in the vaginal, urine, or digestive system);
- unexplained change in bowel habit, bloating, or persistent indigestion;
- any weight loss or gain without apparent explanation; and/or
- difficulty in breathing or swallowing.

Early detection has improved outcomes for several common cancers. At early stage most cancers are treatable and possibly cured.

Early detection saves lives.

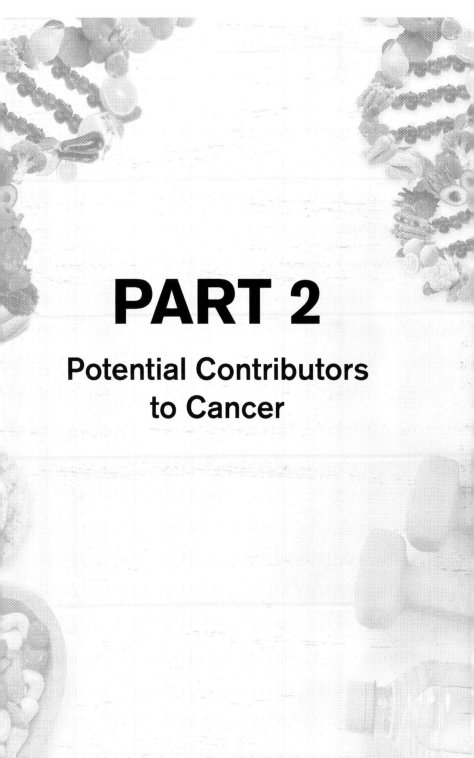

PART 2

Potential Contributors
to Cancer

Chapter 10

Sleep

Sleep, Immune System, and Cancer Risk

Do you toss and turn at night? Do you have difficulties in getting to sleep, staying asleep or both? Do you sleep too little or too much?

If the answer is yes, then you are part of the troubling statistics. An estimated 70 million adults in the United States suffer from a sleep disorder. Taking your condition lightly is risky.

Sleep disorders are of various types, ranging from insomnia to obstructive sleep apnea (OSA, often indicated by heavy snoring). The latter is a condition in which the human body is temporarily deprived of adequate oxygen supply to the blood, i.e., a sleep-related breathing disorder. Sleep deprivation is increasingly common in modern life and results in a predisposition to many disorders.

Modern science backs up the idea that we need a sufficient amount of deep sleep, especially when insufficient sleep can suppress your immune system. Sleep deprivation has a powerful influence on the risk of infectious diseases, the prevalence of depression, the occurrence and progression of major illnesses including cardiovascular disease and cancer.[87-91]

HUI XIE-ZUKAUSKAS, PhD

What your cells do when your body is at rest—an immunity perspective

Sleep is a physiological process, just like breathing and eating—an essential part of the daily life cycle. It is also a key factor for supporting a functional defense system in the body. The human immune system plays a vital role in protecting our bodies from the development of cancer. The cells of our immune systems are our defenders, constantly destroying and eliminating any cell that initiates or undergoes a malignant change. When this natural defense mechanism is weakened, cancerous growth occurs as malignant cells proliferate and then overpower the immune system.

At a cellular level, cytokines, as a critical group of protein players, are involved in the sleep-immune interaction. During deep sleep our bodies work to strengthen our immune system by producing and releasing potent immune-enhancing cytokines. In contrast, cancer-stimulating cytokines may be switched to dominance when sleep is deprived. Particularly, serious sleep disorders (such as OSA) may enhance the proliferative and invasive properties of solid tumors. Collectively, alterations in immune functions trigger the detrimental effects of sleep disorders on cancer development.[88-90]

Emerging evidence points to the association of sleep disturbance and cancer risk. When one is deprived of sleep, the immune T-cell populations go down, and the levels of inflammatory cytokines go up. The inflammatory cytokines, such as IL-1, IL-6, and TNF-α have proven to be a significant contributor to sleep disturbance. Moreover, sleep deficiency can lead to a higher level of C-reactive protein (CRP), an inflammation marker closely linked to cardiovascular diseases. These changes cause escalated inflammation and overwhelmed body defense.

Sleep deprivation can also promote ROS production and oxidative DNA damage.[89] OSA, explicitly intermittent hypoxia and sleep fragmentation, may foster changes in the tumor microenvironment that ultimately lead to a disadvantageous immunosurveillance, thereby accelerating tumor progression and its invasion.[90, 91]

When your immune system is weak and functioning poorly, germs or pathogens can easily penetrate your body and commit destruction to targeted tissues or cells, which is why you are susceptible to cold, flu, and infections. Lack of sleep can also affect how fast your recover if you get sick. In the long-term, sleep deprivation elevates your risk for obesity, diabetes, cardiovascular diseases, neurocognitive impairment, and other severe illnesses.

More facts and findings

Let's look at how sleep may have an impact of sleep on cancer risk and overall health.

1. A little sleep and too much sleep are both associated with higher mortality from all causes of illnesses.
2. Working night shifts with long exposure to light at night disrupts circadian rhythms and has been found to contribute to an increased risk of breast cancer.
3. Patients with OSA have a higher prevalence of cancer and cancer-related death than those without OSA, suggesting that OSA promotes cancer initiation and progression.
4. People living a sedentary lifestyle (i.e., sleeping less than seven hours a day and only participating in moderate to vigorous physical activity less than one hour a week and viewing television more than three hours a day, and also with a BMI greater than twenty-five) had greater episodes of cardiovascular disease and cancer mortality.[92]

5. Individuals with a sleeping disorder are more likely to suffer from chronic conditions such as depression, hypertension, diabetes, obesity, and cancer.
6. Sleep disturbance is among the top ten major health issues in menopausal women.
7. Sleep disturbance or sleep deprivation can critically harm your health based on a reciprocal link between sleep and inflammatory biology. Sleep disorders can adversely affect your immune functions.

In summary, a vast body of data have established that getting adequate sleep has a significant influence on your well-being, especially making your immune system stronger and keeping cancer at bay. On the other hand, insufficient sleep can negatively impact not only health and fitness but also happiness, career, safety, and quality of life.

How to Optimize Your Sleep

A good night's sleep is a good investment in your well-being and productivity. There are various ways to enhance the quality of your sleep (e.g., healthy lifestyle, exercise, stress relief, pain management, as well as pharmacological interventions if necessary). However, sleep hygiene is one of the fundamentals, and you can gain a direct or instant benefit.

That is why I'd prefer a route other than pharmacological management, and specifically recommend a simple and memorable sleep regimen to assist you with optimizing your sleep. This routine uses the acronym ROOM.

Here is how it works.

R is for resting, relaxing, and having a ritual to unwind before bedtime.

O is for zero, referring to zero distraction. Consider distractions ranging from electronic or mobile devices, TV, radio, and bright lights to noises, air, and temperature (an important yet overlooked factor). Eliminate or minimize these interferences from your night environment.

O is for zero again, but this time it refers to zero foods or stimulants. Make sure you don't eat any meal, especially a big meal, two hours prior to your bedtime. Avoid alcohol, coffee, sugary drinks, or any stimulant medication. Limit water intake too in order to curtail unnecessary bathroom trips.

M is for mandating the time and mattress. This is crucial to ensure your full sleep time—seven to eight hours per night for an adult. To achieve this, go to bed and wake up at the same time every day. Stick with this routine even during the weekends. Remember to buy a really good and comfortable mattress. It's worth it.

Equally important is to find out the causes of your sleeping problem, and don't rely on sleeping pills unless drug intervention becomes absolutely necessary.

If you still have trouble sleeping, it's paramount to seek professional help to determine any underlying psychological or pathophysiological issue.

At the end of the day, adequate duration and good quality of sleep can definitely go a long way toward securing your optimal health, a lowered cancer risk, and enhanced vitality. Because getting enough sleep is very valuable for your overall wellness, make the most of it!

I hope you sleep like a baby and smile like a baby too.

Chapter 11 ——————————————

Stress

Stress and Cancer Risk

Have you ever been stressed? I raise my hand first.

Stress is unavoidable and undeniable, though its magnitude can vary. Life stress may come from the death of a loved one, illnesses, divorce, debt, and job loss. It could even come down to a parking fine, daily traffic jams, a conflict with someone, or just a bad day at work. Depending on the situation, you may experience grief, anxiety, concern, depression, fear, frustration, or anger. After all, we all know what it's like to feel stress.

Stress seems mental, but it's not just mental or psychological. Mental stress can translate into physical changes in the body as many of us have experienced. Chronic or persisted stress can make you sick.

How can stress contribute to cancer risk and heart disease?

The direct effect of stress on cancer risk or cancer development still remains unclear. However, considerable scientific research has found out how psychological stress can change the human body in various ways.[93-96]

Stress can increase inflammation.

Studies reveal that elevated levels of CRP, a biomarker of inflammation, occur when individuals engage in stressful situations. Prolonged stress and negative emotions alter normal immune responses, resulting in the production and release of pro-inflammatory chemicals that trigger inflammation instead of regulating inflammation properly. Inflammation plays a central role in many chronic conditions, such as initiating cardiovascular disease and promoting cancer development.

Stress can facilitate the production of free radicals.

Stress is responsible for generating free radicals. As established, various carcinogens exert their effects partly via the production of ROS. Endogenous free radicals generated from cellular metabolism may participate in chronic inflammation, diabetes, viral infection and aging process through oxidative injury. Moreover, stress hormone signaling pathways may cause DNA damage through producing ROS and interfering DNA repair process, leading to carcinogenesis.

Stress can promote immune dysfunction.

The immune system is a critical element when it comes to intensifying, preventing, and treating chronic illnesses, but the stress from everyday life may significantly bring down its functions. Chronic stress or depression can increase the production of cytokines, and one of them is IL-6. High levels of IL-6 have been associated with an increased risk for several adverse conditions, such as cardiovascular disease, type 2 diabetes, some types of cancers, and mental health problems. In a plain term, IL-6 acts as an immune modulating agent, which is also a product of bad mood. It can negatively impact the immune system.

Stress can cause weight gain.

Stress hormones stimulate a craving for foods rich in sugar, fat, and starch. Does that sound familiar? That's so-called stress eating. Psychological stress affects eating through the effect of cortisol and brain reward circuit on calorie-dense food intake. Stress and palatable food (e.g., sweets) can stimulate endogenous opioid release and cause the feeling of euphoria or experience of self-indulging, which in turn may serve as a robust defense against stress.[97] As a result, high calories from junk food and pleasant eating add extra pounds over time. The stress response may also bring a rise in circulating insulin and a fall in fat oxidation (i.e., fat burning), and it tends to increase abdominal fat storage. So a complex yet delicate link between stress and weight gain may arise from poor eating habits under stress.

Stress is a contributor to the progression of various illnesses.

Stress is connected with psychological or emotional components (e.g., depression, anxiety, and anger). Their intensity has an adverse impact on cancer incidence or survival and the development of heart disease as well. Various studies suggest that chronic stress is a primary source of more than 95 percent of all clinical conditions.

Overall, the relationship between stress and cancer is intricate. Many factors come into play. However, chronic stress is linked to the six leading causes of death—heart disease, cancer, lung ailments, accidents, suicide, and liver cirrhosis.

Stress cycle

As mentioned previously, many folks who are stressed out end up eating, drinking, and smoking more but exercising less. Subsequently, these unhealthy behaviors worsen the tough condition. All products of bad mood, together with additional stressors or pathogens, can lead to amplified or prolonged inflammatory responses that aggravate a harmful cycle or sequence of stress.

Stress can also exacerbate sleep deficits. In turn, people with troubled sleep often find it hard to deal with the stress in their lives.

As a vicious cycle, stress really imposes chaos on both the mind and the body. Therefore, managing stress is a must for you to live a healthy, long, and productive life.

Your tool-box

Here are eleven effective strategies and tips to combat, reduce, or minimize stress.

1. **Practice gratitude, and maintain a positive attitude.**

    Gratitude is the foundation of our day-to-day happiness. So commit to appreciating small, simple things and other things we often take for granted, such as sunny days or good health. I believe that my gratitude practice each morning is a profoundly effective routine that helps me maintain a positive, joyful mind-set for the rest of the day and push through challenging times as well. Likewise, a gratitude journal (e.g., writing in it for approximately five minutes a day), a thank-you card, and small acts to return kindness all nurture the quality of being thankful.

To tune in high spirits, start off your day with gratitude, not on social media.

2. Ensure sufficient and restful sleep.

Having at least seven to eight hours of sleep a night is essential for a relaxed body and mind. Plus, you reap the benefits of a less stressful day ahead of you. When you're well rested, it's much easier to concentrate with a clear mind, solve problems, and optimize productivity. Also, you likely become less grumpy, irritated, or frustrated. Ironically, stress can cause sleepless nights, as you likely end up worrying while staring at the ceiling. So sleep healthily, with the help of ROOM regimen (in the Chapter on Sleep).

3. Identify a trigger or stressor, and find the solutions for it.

Numerous factors can cause stress. So what may be yours? Next, retrace, recall, and dig deeper within yourself honestly to uncover those triggers. Then use all your senses (i.e., sight, smell, sound, taste, and touch) to find the best solutions to your problem.

4. Exercise, exercise, and exercise.

Exercises are a great stress reliever. It offers huge yet cost-effective benefits for better sleep and less stress. There are so many practical ways to do so. For example, take a long walk at a park or a short one around the neighborhood. Join a group class for yoga or do yoga at home. Find a location with no strain from time or weather. It's even greater if you can start biking, running, jogging, swimming, or jumping rope in the backyard.

5. Create your unique stress-relief techniques.

It could be soothing music, a workout at the gym, meditation, a relaxing massage, or a weekend getaway. It could also come with things as simple as deep breathing, a hot bath, or playing with kids. Whatever works for you, practice it. Because your stress is unique to your matter and thus, so is your solution. It's better to create and experience your own workable techniques (e.g., an outdoor yoga practice, lunch with a friend, or a visit to the museum), notably those that combine a hobby with being physically active.

6. Have fun and a sense of humor even if you feel hopeless or powerless.

Try to take your mind off your problem. Humor and fun can be your formula. Remember that laughter is your best medicine and effective coping mechanism for stress. Yes, laughter can trigger the release of feel-good endorphins— the body's natural pain reliever or happiness booster.

7. Keep a balanced diet.

Diet factors (e.g., poor diet, malnutrition, and food allergies) can play a substantial part in mental and emotional difficulties. Restrain from certain items (e.g., alcohol, cigarettes, or coffee) of personal preference for stress relief, because they can make your stress bigger or worse and potentially destroy your health. So eat well, and eat a lot of nutrient-rich foods.

8. **Unplug by applying a screen-smart solution (i.e., digital detox).**

We are in a digital age, and convenience comes with a price. Internet and smartphone addictions have become a real and serious problem because endless texting and emails affect the health, life, and social connections of many people, especially kids. Without doubt, this is a stressor or stress enabler.

To relieve stress, you can curb or control your screen time. Don't keep your iPhone or iPad in your bedroom next to your pillow. Minimize the times and/or period you check email or text messages, and limit the time you spend on Facebook, Twitter, or other social platforms. By making a smart decision about screen time, you can make more time for your family or friends and keep yourself calm.

9. **Choose your priorities and set realistic expectations.**

If you have trouble with time management or saying no, it's time to set a priority for the most important and urgent things at work or off work. Avoid putting things off, as procrastination can paradoxically be the root of anxiety and stress. So pick your battles without self-doubt.

10. **Connect to a network of support and enhance your overall well-being.**

Mental or emotional wellness is not separated from other areas of your life. Have a social network of care and support to counter depression and isolation. At the same time, preserve and enhance various areas of your well-being, including your family's well-being, career well-being, financial well-being, and relationship well-being.

11. Show love and compassion to someone else or a great cause.

Think less about yourself for a while. Shift your focus away from the pain, and look at the bigger picture. Doing so can be helpful and rewarding. There are numerous inspirational stories on coming out of extremely stressful situations.

Gratitude Note

I'm not implying that everybody should show gratitude equally, and I'm not considering such without empathy for those people who have unjustly or chronically suffered from staggering illnesses. I acknowledge that there is no way to spin profound personal loss or staggering severe illnesses.

Coping with Stress during Holidays

Although stress can affect all aspects of our lives, stress means different things to different people. What causes stress in one person may be of little concern to another. Let me engage in how to better cope with holiday stress, as many folks can relate to it.

The holiday season can be both joyful and overwhelmingly stressful. Yes, the festive holiday season is full of beauty, bliss, love, and excitement. But do you know that one of the clinical triggers of heart attack includes holidays like Christmas and New Year's Day? Various factors play a role, and emotional stress is one.

Others such as overindulgence, unchecked chronic conditions, and weight gain—all put extra stress on a weakened heart too. Accumulated findings have confirmed that stress management can reduce your risk.

Holiday stress can come in diverse forms and at different levels. What do they look like?

Holiday realities

Stress is a facet of holiday norms. Besides our usual workload and family commitment, we have new functions or activities as we rush around trying to meet looming deadlines. There are more parties, social events, holiday shopping, decorating, going to watch new movies, and entertaining the guests. Oh, and wait a minute. What about holiday meals and trips out of town? See how much we try to cram into the festive season! It gives me a headache just naming these things.

Now imagine doing all that. It's certainly a recipe for stress. No wonder many people are stressed out.

How do you survive holiday stress and enjoy a happy time?

The true happiness or glory of the holiday season is found in our hearts—not in the malls, at the parties, or from luxurious gifts.

First, understand your needs versus your stress.

Holiday stress normally falls into categories of financial, physical, psychological, or emotional drains. So acknowledge your feelings. Putting things in perspective and realistically assessing your needs can ease your burden considerably, and also help you prevent depression.

There are times during the holidays when things seem to go wrong. It may feel as if there's too much to do and not enough time. When you feel overwhelmed by the dos, you should set priorities and keep the following prime points in mind:

- Material items or gifts might bring you a moment of sensation and joy, but they cannot fulfill your inner peace and happiness in the long run.
- Meeting social obligations and outside expectations might seem important, but it can't replace your time for family, friends, and loved ones.
- You can find happiness and contentment by adjusting your standards or unrealistic desires and selecting satisfactory alternatives. Refocus on what you have instead of what you don't have.

Win control over stress with these ten power bonuses.

1. **Plan ahead based on PBS. Prioritize, be realistic, and simplify.**

   Planning involves what activities you may do and what to skip, what and who is on your shopping list, when to shop, what are on your meal menus, and so on. Learn to say no. Don't let yes overthrow you.

2. **Take it easy.**

   Make the holidays pleasant rather than perfect. If a card cannot get to its destination on time, give the person a surprise call on that holiday morning! If you don't feel like cooking or baking, buy some ready meals as an alternative, or go without one or two traditions. Instead of spending hours at the mall or sitting in traffic, shop online for gifts. You could get better deals that way too.

3. **Tap the resources within your family or from neighbors and friends.**

   Delegate some tasks. If you love decorating the tree but hate dishwashing, trade cleaning up with other family members. Make sure that everybody gets to pick his or her favorites or take turns. For meals, a potluck is always fun.

4. **Stick to a budget within your means.**

   If you're on a tight budget but your holiday gift list keeps growing, just buy small items. Plus we all can be creative in a way to spend less or give thoughtful presents that money can't buy. Most people appreciate any gift regardless of its size. Alternatively, you can initiate a gift-free holiday. Just make sure you let people know early. If it's too costly to attend a fancy party, organize a novel yet fun activity to celebrate at home. By spending wisely, you'll avoid new-year depression because of debt.

5. **Listen to your body and make time for yourself.**

   If you are tired, rest. If you crave a treat or massage, get it, and if you need a regular workout, go for it. If all you want is some quiet downtime or a nap, allow yourself that.

6. **Practice stress-relieving techniques that particularly work for you.**

   Just because the letters in *desserts* can be used to spell *stressed*, that doesn't mean you can relieve stress with desserts. Take caution with high-sugar and high-calorie foods. Instead, breathe deeply, meditate freely, visualize a peaceful scene, or listen to soothing and relaxing music.

7. **Mind healthy habits.**

Overdrinking, overeating, and more sedentary behavior can aggravate stress. They can even lead to adverse consequences. When the unexpected happens, it adds stress to the folks around you.

8. **Laugh, laugh, and laugh more!**

Laughter is a powerful medicine. Find humor or something (e.g., watching a comedy) to laugh about! It's scientifically and clinically proven that laughter decreases circulating levels of stress hormones and increases the release of stress-relieving endorphins. Laughter has a positive influence on heart rate, blood pressure, lung capacity, musculoskeletal system and brain activity, thereby promoting overall health.

9. **The holiday season is a time for family, friends, and fun!**

This is perhaps the most important tip of all! Connecting with people you love and having fun gathering can be the most effective stress reliever and immune booster. Keep in mind that this is a time of loneliness and depression for some. So invite them to your home, and offer kindness to them. On the other hand, if you are alone, reaching out to help others can benefit your own physical and psychological well-being.

10. **Pay special attention to the caregivers.** They also deserve our gratitude and care.

Remember that spending time with family and friends and having fun will turn the holiday frenzy into holiday bliss!

And let the season's joy boost your immune system.

It isn't what you have, who you are, where you are, what you are doing that makes you happy or unhappy; It is what you think about.

—Dale Carnegie

Chapter 12

Substance Abuse

Substance Misuse or Abuse and Cancer Risk

The blessings of narcotic painkillers or opioid analgesics for therapeutic usage are beyond doubt. However, the misuse or abuse of illicit/illegal drugs and prescription medications poses a threat to public health.

Opioids have become the cornerstone of cancer pain management. There is also a rapid increase in opioid prescriptions in an effort to address the growing health problem of chronic pain. Illicit drug overdose has led to increasing addictions and deaths. Unfortunately, amid the opioid crisis, all constitute grave concerns and affect the well-being of millions of people.

Yes, substance abuse increases cancer risk and some of cancer incidents.[98, 99] Specifically, opium use has been associated with an increased risk for cancers of the upper aerodigestive tract and bladder.[100, 101] Substance abuse is a clearly preventable contributor to cancer.

How substance abuse can increase cancer risk

Substance abuse takes various forms, including tobacco, alcohol, and drugs. Tobacco products, especially cigarettes, contain more than seventy known carcinogens. Similarly, alcohol intake is linked to several types of cancer and there is no safe level for alcohol consumption as to cancer risk. Some substances such as marijuana, heroin, cocaine, and steroids present a different risk for the development of cancer. Nevertheless, the carcinogens found in tobacco are also concentrated in marijuana.

Chronic substance abuse plays a role in the pathogenesis of cancer. Although a direct relationship between substance abuse and cancer risk is not strongly established, research data indicates that drug abuse can participate in the process of cancer development through the mutagenic effects of certain substances and a dysregulated immune system.[98-100]

Furthermore, other factors including lifestyle may influence one's cancer risk, which is the possibility that a clear causal mechanism is not always well defined. For instance, some individuals with the problem of substance abuse often engage in other risky behaviors such as tobacco and/or alcohol use, and the latter can cause many types of cancer.

Since tobacco smoking and alcohol consumption have been covered in previous chapters, here we shall discuss more about some illicit drugs.

Steroids

Anabolic steroids are manufactured products that perform like the male hormone testosterone. They are linked to a number of adverse outcomes, including cancer, organ damage and a higher risk for HIV and hepatitis because of health hazard from sharing needles for injection.[102, 103]

The liver is the primary organ responsible for metabolizing and clearing out chemicals (e.g., drugs, steroids) from the blood. Accumulated steroid abuse can cause liver damage that may lead to liver tumor (i.e., hepatic adenomas, a benign tumor but it can turn cancerous). Disturbingly, the leading causes of liver cancer are hepatitis, chronic alcohol and substance abuse.

Moreover, the effects of steroids on hormonal changes and immune function can elevate the risk for prostate, breast, cervical, and endometrial cancer, and other common cancers of the liver, kidney, pancreas, skin and non-Hodgkin lymphoma.[102, 103]

Opiates, Opioids

Opiates include a variety of drugs ranging from legal ones such as codeine, morphine, and fentanyl to illegal ones such as heroin. Make a note of that opium is a powerful and natural form of opiates and it's commonly smoked by individuals worldwide.

While subtle, the distinction between opioids and opiates is significant. An *opiate* is a drug naturally derived from the flowering opium poppy plant. Examples of opiates include heroin, morphine, and codeine. On the other hand, the name *opioid* is a broader term that includes opiates and refers to any substance, natural or synthetic, that binds to the brain's opioid receptors.

Although all opiates are opioids, *not* all opioids are opiates.

Prescription opioids include codeine, morphine, oxycodone (i.e., OxyContin˚, Percocet˚), and fentanyl. Fentanyl is a powerful, synthetic opioid 50 to 100 times more potent than morphine.

An estimated 16.5 million people worldwide illicitly use opiates, of which 4 million use raw opium. Opioids and/or opiates can be highly addictive and extremely toxic. Studies have found that opioids such as morphine possibly promote cancer growth. Opium use is linked to an increased risk for cancers of the esophagus, stomach, larynx, lung, and bladder.[99-101]

There are different types of narcotic painkillers. Two of the most notorious forms of narcotic drugs are opium and heroin.

Heroin

Heroin, the most abused opiate drug, is a semi-synthetic opiate derived from morphine, and also one of the most dangerous drugs in the world.

Although heroin can be ingested by smoking, snorting, and injecting, injection via veins is the most dangerous and deadliest way, because first, one can easily be overdosed and die; and second, individuals who share insanitary or contaminated needles with other users are at a higher risk for contracting HIV/AIDS or hepatitis.

Long-term heroin abuse may result in lung complications and liver diseases, and may also increase the risk for liver and stomach cancer.[104]

Marijuana (or Cannabis)

There is an increasing concern that marijuana or cannabis smoking may be a risk factor for tobacco-related cancers.[105-111] Marijuana smoke contains PAH and other carcinogens at a higher concentration than tobacco smoke. Marijuana tar contains several of the same carcinogens and toxic chemicals as tobacco smoking. However, each marijuana exposure may be more harmful than a tobacco cigarette since more tar is inhaled and retained when smoking marijuana, which is confirmed by the respiratory abnormalities and oral lesions found in marijuana users compared to nonsmokers.[112] Growing experimental and clinical data show that marijuana smoke is a risk factor for lung cancer.

Marijuana smoking is also associated with a greater risk of head and neck cancer, and the risk increases dose-dependently.[109, 110] One of the components of marijuana is delta-9-tetrahydrocannabinol (THC), a psychoactive substance. THC produces a relaxing or euphoric effect and can relieve pain. But its tumor-promoting properties include suppressing immunity and escalating ROS. Cannabis contains high levels of THC too.

Heavy use of marijuana has been associated with substantial adverse consequences. It causes inflammation of the airway and increases the risk of cardiovascular events such as heart attack, stroke, etc. Some studies show that marijuana smoking induces lung injury with precancerous changes, including increased tar exposure, dysfunctional macrophages on tumor-elimination, intensified oxidative stress, and bronchial mucosa abnormalities. Other findings implicate a link between cannabis use and an elevated risk of bladder and prostate cancer.[113]

Given the prevalence of marijuana smoking, marijuana smokers should take caution to avoid potential adverse health outcomes.

Stimulants

Stimulants such as *cocaine* and prescription stimulants such as *amphetamine* may also raise a risk of developing cancer. They have been particularly associated with an increased risk for the development of non-Hodgkin lymphoma.[99, 114, 115] Notably, cocaine has immunosuppressive effect. Cocaine use is linked to a greater risk of cancer-related HPV infection.[116] Amphetamine may induce DNA damage.[117]

In brief, these drugs or substances possess the capability to cause genotoxicity, potentially contribute to the initiation, promotion and progression of various types of cancer.

Concomitant use of tobacco, alcohol, marijuana or any illicit drug

Any type of smoking habit exposes individuals to a wide range of carcinogens. Alcohol consumption (beer or wine) makes carcinogens such as ethanol and acetaldehyde operative on most of the gastrointestinal tract. Ethanol also acts as a solvent in the oral mucosa and thus enhances the cellular membrane permeability to carcinogens.

Moreover, excess alcohol plays a greater role in drug abuse and remains the primary toxic agent for the liver that hepatitis patients should avoid. Co-abuse of marijuana or psychostimulants with alcohol can increase the risk of developing different types of cancer.[118, 119]

Tobacco use, alcohol consumption and unhealthy lifestyles or risky behaviors are often connected with substance use, and all are genotoxic. So imagine adding all these substances up.

Additional hazards

Most substances of abuse can be consumed in a variety of ways (i.e., smoking, snorting, swallowing, and injection). Injection is the riskiest and most dangerous delivery method. Injecting drugs with contaminated needles is a well-known route of HIV exposure and viral hepatitis transmission.

There is also production exposure because illegal substances often contain carcinogenic additives. Many chemicals used in manufacturing illicit substances are toxic or carcinogen. So individuals are exposed to chemical pollution or contamination during production. Likewise, in a case of improper disposal, the materials or wastes can put people and communities nearby in a harmful condition.

Cancer is a prime threat for long-term substance abuse, in addition to neuropsychological damage. For cancer treatment, substance abuse can reduce treatment compliance, worsen cancer prognosis, and negatively impact the quality of life among these cancer patients.

Taken together, chronic substance abuse can lead to numerous health consequences, including an increased risk for the development and progression of cancer. Again, substance abuse is a preventable contributor to cancer!

A final and sensible note

I am fully aware and understand that many addictions grow from reliance on painkillers prescribed for a health issue, a treatment of postsurgical pain, or severe and unbearable chronic pain. You should not discontinue your treatment on pain relief.

On the other hand, the opioid epidemic and addiction also involve the ingestion of powerful painkillers overprescribed by physicians. Clinical guidelines should be reexamined and reinforced, but that is beyond the scope of this book.

However, it is of critical importance to know three key points before taking a narcotic painkiller:

- First, painkillers don't cure your disease. All they do is to relieve the pain.
- Second, these painkillers produce momentary or short-term euphoria that can be highly addictive, but long-term usage can lead to physical dependence.
- Finally, respiratory depression or collapse is one of the fatal risks of opioids and powerful painkillers. In particular, the drugs cause the user's breathing to slow down and then to stop eventually (i.e., respiratory arrest and death), which can happen at high dosages or with the intake of alcohol and other drugs together (e.g., barbiturates and certain benzodiazepines).

For people who have to depend on prescription pain medications, here are five valued strategies for managing your intake.

1. *Understand the nature of these painkillers, especially therapeutic effects and side effects.* Remember that a drug's side effects are not your fault. But being aware of any signs of addiction or physical dependence is your choice. It is in your power to control your habits.

2. *Discuss symptoms of withdrawal, curbing the duration of treatment, or alternative treatment plan with your physician.*

3. *Recognize the misuse.* Misuses range from taking an extra dosage or extending the duration beyond your prescription to taking other people's prescriptions, etc. Substance abuse is a chronic disorder too, so you want to prevent it without adding to your existing health issue.

4. *If you encounter an overdose, treat with naloxone, a fast-acting antidote for opioid overdoses.* Remember that treatment is always there for you, so get it.

5. *Seek professional help and treatment.* Don't hesitate. For people suffering from an addiction disorder, it's crucial that you do not stigmatize your condition.

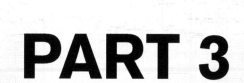

PART 3

Specific Risk Factors for Most Common and Malignant Cancers

Chapter 13 ——————————

Breast Cancer

B reast cancer is the most common female cancer worldwide, the second most common cancer and the second leading cause of cancer deaths among women in the United States after lung cancer.

The potential causes of breast cancer include genetic predisposition, alcohol consumption, environmental pollutants, lifestyle factors, and long-term HRT.

Risk factors can be divided into modifiable and unmodifiable risk factors. There are also differences between pre- and post-menopausal breast cancer, particularly regarding risk factors. It should be noted that menopause itself does not cause cancer, but the risk of developing cancer increases as a woman is aging.

Modifiable risk factors include

- pregnancy history (never giving birth or pregnancy at late ages),
- not breast-feeding,
- use of birth control pills,
- hormone therapy after menopause,
- environmental toxins (especially endocrine-disrupting chemicals)
- frequent alcohol consumption,

- obesity (especially overweight or obese after menopause),
- lack of physical activity, and
- induced abortion.

Unmodifiable risk factors include

- gender,
- age (getting older),
- genetic mutations,
- family history or personal history of breast cancer,
- personal history of certain non-cancerous breast conditions,
- dense breast tissue,
- menstrual periods (i.e., early menstruation or menopause after age fifty-five),
- breast radiation early in life, and
- chemotherapy.

Although many risk factors may increase the chance of developing breast cancer, being well informed and early detection can save lives considerably. However, common barriers or problems still exist, including late presentation of symptoms for medical attention and delayed diagnosis resulting from care systems, especially in developing countries or economically poor populations where early screening is not accessible.

That's why breast cancer awareness and prevention should use multiple approaches. It's imperative to do things beyond wearing pink in October each year.

We must consider the following topics or areas:

- genetic aspect with energy view
- daily risk factors for everybody (because men get breast cancer too)

- five estrogen sources (because more and longer exposure to this hormone increases the risk of breast cancer)
- early detection (because breast cancer prevention is for everyone)

The Genetics and Energy View of Breast Cancer Prevention

I'd like to focus on two factors related to breast cancer—genetics and energy.

Let me start with breast cancer genes BRCA1 and BRCA2 (signaling an abbreviation for BReast CAncer). I'm going to use a simple diagram here to illustrate how a mutation of BRCA genes is linked to breast cancer.

Schematic Illustration 4. BRCA genes and their roles

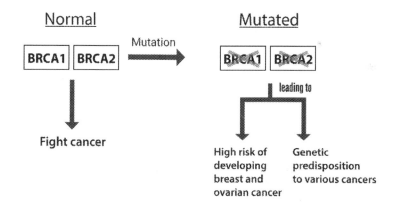

BRCA1 and BRCA2 genes are cancer suppressors. Their function is to protect a cell from developing cancer, thereby helping you fight or prevent cancer. When either of these genes becomes mutated (i.e., modified in a harmful way), that gene no longer functions properly. As a result of unrepaired DNA damage and impaired genetic integrity, the cells are more likely to grow uncontrollably and develop into cancer (like a car racing on the highway without brakes).

We all have BRCA1 and BRCA2 genes, both women and men, because BRCA is not a sex-linked gene. The mutation can be inherited from either parent. For women with a BRCA mutation, the lifetime risk of breast cancer is approximately 80 percent, and the chance of ovarian cancer is 54 percent. Men may carry the BRCA mutation, but they have a lower risk.

However, the genes do not tell the full story. Of more than 200,000 breast cancer cases newly diagnosed each year, BRCA gene mutation accounts for about 10 percent of them. And the fact is that about 85 percent of women diagnosed with breast cancer have no family history of the disease.[120] Thus, there is one or more promising areas for treatment and prevention.

Among guiding philosophies of traditional Chinese medicine (TCM), the holistic health system urges one to prevent diseases rather than just treat them. A treasured remedy for cancer prevention is to safeguard against a holistic imbalance resulting from poor diet, unhealthy lifestyle, harmful stressors or environmental pollutions, and to strengthen your inner qi.

Now let me dive a little deeper into qi (vital energy).

As we conversed previously, qi is the vital energy that moves with blood throughout the body at all times. It is everywhere in the body and interconnected with the organs, which keeps our wholeness in balance. Stagnation of flowing qi and blood over time leads to mass, lump or tumor.

What can cause qi stagnation?

In TCM's view, one of the causes for qi stagnation is attributed to emotional imbalance. Specifically, when intensive, persistent emotions dominate (e.g., uncontrolled anger, depression or lasting grief), not only can they interrupt normal harmony of organ functions, but also they impair the immune system. For example, according to TCM, *anger hurts the liver, overexcitement hurts the heart, anxiety hurts the spleen, grief hurts the lung, and fear hurts the kidney.* So, one of diseases for which there is a great concern about the adverse effect of emotional distress or disturbance is cancer.

In essence, this notion is comparable with Western medicine on the role of psychological or psychosocial factors in some diseases. Particularly, psychological stress may impact breast cancer onset and progression.[121] Clearly, emotions do not automatically modify the genes, but they do trigger a surge of cellular changes that affect the immunity and alter the genes associated with stress.

Together, the human body is susceptible to cancer when it's under emotional stress or trauma. Hence, strategies and activities that control emotions should be among the valuable pursuits in strengthening qi and sustaining health.

How can we harness vital and healing energy to prevent cancer?

Here are eight ways.

1. **Make your immune system strong**. Our immune system is our powerhouse to fight cancer. That's why scientific innovations tap into the body's immune system to destroy cancer cells. When cancer overwhelms your body's immune capacity and healing power, it leads to a tragic ending. So, cultivate healing energy through strong immunity.

2. **Control your emotions to keep qi flow.** Maintaining a positive outlook on life helps boost your positive energy. Anger, fear, sadness, and anxiety can adversely affect your

qi. Have you noticed that stress can drain your energy? Conversely, joy, happiness, and the harmony between emotions and organs can build up your vibrant qi. Another key to flowing qi is to share your feeling, let it out and let it go.

3. **Foster gratitude.** Devote time (at least a few minutes a day) to appreciate what you have, even the small things. Keep content, cheerful, and compassionate. Doing so will help channel your enlightened spirit and vital energy!

4. **Go for a nutrient-packed diet.** Various factors of food (including quantity, quality, cooking or processing) influence qi, so be aware of them. Nutrition supports both the level and the quality of your energy. A balanced diet with plenty of fruits, vegetables, proteins and whole grains but limited fats and alcohol can prevent qi deficiency.

5. **Exercise regularly and purposely.** Be physically active because it keeps qi moving and blood circulating! In addition, exercises such as Qigong and Yoga involve both movement and mindfulness. Mindfulness is to stay in the moment and to avoid distractions from unwanted thoughts or external stimuli. Intentionally practice the moves that you love, and practice deep breathing or meditation to elevate your inner awareness.

6. **Maintain a healthy weight.** Obesity is a state of energy imbalance and a noteworthy risk factor of breast cancer. It is partly related to sluggish qi and metabolic dysfunction. Healthy weight plays a critical role in lowering the risks of cancer growth and cancer recurrence.

7. **Rest and relax well.** Sufficient sleep can restore vibrant qi, cultivate healing qi, and maintain the holistic harmony.

8. **Be vigilant about early detection!** Get a genetic screening to identify the BRCA gene mutation, and start effective measure or therapy early. Treat any illness early. Doing so will help protect your vital energy.

Breast cancer prevention is for both women and men, and it is based on our shared genetics. We cannot control our genes, gender, age, race, or family history. However, each and every one of us can strengthen our qi and foster a healthy lifestyle, which is vital to staying healthy and keeping cancer at bay.

Daily Risks for Breast Cancer: Everybody Can Do Something

Why everybody? Because both men and women can get breast cancer and because you care about your loved ones, you can join the fight for a great cause.

Unless you have a well-defined plan, here is food for thought.

In addition to wearing pink (clothing or a ribbon) in honor of those who are currently fighting breast cancer and/or who died of breast cancer, campaigning to raise funds for research and getting a mammogram for early detection, there are fundamental things that everybody can do in every October and all year.

First of all, the key to fighting breast cancer is to catch it early, which will be addressed later on.

Then the best cure is prevention.

DNA mutation can occur over one's lifetime. That's excluding inheritance from one's family. That's why lowering your risk for breast cancer is important. Did you know that about 85 percent of women diagnosed with breast cancer have no family history of the disease?

Again, you cannot control family history and/or genetics, but you can surely avoid or minimize your exposure to factors that cause DNA mutation.

What are five most common daily risks for breast cancer?

These include

1. smoking,
2. drinking alcohol,
3. eating junk foods (processed foods and food low in nutrients but high in fat, sugar, and salt),
4. inhaling or ingesting environmental pollutants and toxins, and
5. being physically inactive.

Everybody can relate to these health hazards, right? Be aware that some of them are hidden. Of course, there are other risk factors for breast cancer, including hormone therapy, radiation, sleeping pattern (night shift), and aging. Certainly, the latter cannot be modified in a biological sense.

To be clear, it's not one single factor that plays a measurable role in causing any cancer. Multiple factors impact the development of breast cancer too. For instance, when combined with genetic factors, alcohol consumption and cigarette smoking enhance a risk for breast cancer and several other cancers as well. Likewise, our environment can influence our genes. There is sharp distinction between the genetic factors we cannot control and environmental or lifestyle ones that we can.

Furthermore, each cancer is different. No two people have the exactly same cancer.

How can you reduce your risk of breast cancer?

Breast cancer prevention starts with a healthy lifestyle, such as stopping tobacco usage, limiting alcohol consumption, getting a nutritious diet, staying physically active, keeping a healthy weight, and avoiding environmental toxins if you can. Lifestyle modification is often most effective and can go a long way.

Lifestyle change doesn't happen overnight. It often works by taking small, simple steps on a daily basis to make an incremental progress. Just consider food. Eating a diet rich in fruits, vegetables, and abundant nutrients, but low in fat and sugar, has been shown to help fight breast cancer. Every meal counts. Plus eating well can facilitate a healthy weight and decrease your risk for several other types of cancer.

Regular physical activities also offer you protective benefits. Research has demonstrated that women who exercised vigorously or moderately were significantly less risky to get breast cancer compared with those who didn't exercise. Getting physically active further support a peaceful mind and a restful sleep, and better emotional health.

Healthy eating and active living, together with an eco-friendly, sustainable environment, have a great potential to lower obesity prevalence, breast cancer risk and incidence.

Five Estrogen Sources and Breast Cancer Risk

As mentioned earlier, hormones play a role in the development of breast cancer. Because longer exposure to estrogen increases a woman's risk of breast cancers, some ignored or forgotten concerns need to be addressed.

Estrogen is a steroid hormone made from cholesterol, and it occurs in both women and men. It promotes the growth and development of sex organs and reproductive tissues. However, too much estrogen can have other effects. In fact, it can increase a risk of cancer. Specifically, a body of data confirm that elevated levels of estrogen have been linked to breast cancer. Estrogen steers the development of breast cancer through its ability to stimulate proliferation and inhibit fatality of cancerous cells.[122]

Having said that, do you know how much unwanted estrogens—some of which are toxic—are around in our modern society? That's why I direct your attention to their sources.

There are five major sources of uninvited estrogen—foods, physical inactivity, obesity, environmental toxins, and HRT.

Let me go over them one by one and help you adopt strategies to eliminate excess estrogen from your daily life.

Poor diet and unhealthy foods

Without a doubt, synthetic hormone-containing foods are available everywhere. For example, a lot of beef and dairy products are pumped up with synthetic growth hormones that can interrupt your hormone balance if you often consume them. Excess carbohydrates from refined foods and sugar are normally not needed for energy, so if you eat a lot, they will be stored as fat in your body. Read on to find out what happens next.

Obesity

Obesity is a significant lifestyle factor related to cancer risk. Obesity is also an established risk factor for breast cancer especially in postmenopausal women, and for developing estrogen-driven breast cancer. Think about this.

Obesity is the source of chronic inflammation of white adipose tissue, and it has been associated with an abnormally high level of aromatase, an enzyme responsible for estrogen production by converting testosterone to estrogen. Research in postmenopausal women also indicates that obese individuals tend to have higher estrogen levels than their lean counterparts.

So the fatty tissue is one of the factories that produce estrogen in the body. As a result, obesity fueled aromatase in the breast and elevated local estrogen formation increase the susceptibility to breast cancer development.

Lack of exercise

Living a sedentary lifestyle is closely associated with obesity and hormone imbalance. Strong evidence suggests that exercise can regulate the balance of estrogen. Thus, a lack of exercise can cause estrogen accumulation in the body.

Environmental toxins

Xenoestrogens—many call these "fake estrogens" or man-made toxins—are a group of chemicals present in the environment and everyday products. They mimic the effects of estrogen in your body.[59] When excessive estrogen accumulates in the body, normal hormone functions are compromised.

Xenoestrogens are often present in

- household cleaners;
- household plastics products (e.g., plastic containers and bottles);
- personal care products (e.g., nail polish and nail polish removers);
- pesticides, fungicides, or herbicides; and
- industrial pollutants.

Hormone replacement therapy (HRT) and birth control pills

Estrogen and progesterone are naturally occurring hormones. Although women (younger than 60 years old) can benefit from HRT for menopause-related symptoms, clinical studies also reveal that HRT can increase the risks for breast cancer, cardiovascular events, heart attack, and stroke. Likewise, synthetic hormones such as estrogen are used in birth control pills. Research shows that the earlier a girl begins to use contraceptives, the greater her risk of breast cancer is.

Collectively, because estrogen is a major hormonal contributor to breast cancer risk, the sources or factors that alter the hormone levels can have a substantial impact.

In essence, overloaded estrogen in your body may come from the food you eat, the amount of exercise you get, the weight you carry, the place you live and work, and possibly the drugs you take. Elevated estrogen can impact not only breast cancer but also other cancers. Furthermore, the next generations may be impacted severely because their exposure during early life leads to illnesses later. Therefore, prevent excess estrogens from sneaking into your body.

Detect Early and Catch Early

To save lives, the most important factor is catching cancer early. At an early stage, cancer is mostly treatable. And if you're at a higher risk for cancer, it can be closely monitored.

You can go deeper to the root of cancer too. Let's start with people who are most vulnerable to the risk posed by BRCA gene mutations. A mutation of BRCA genes has been a causal link to breast cancer. Indeed, a harmful BRCA1 or BRCA2 mutation can be inherited from a person's mother or father. Thus, BRCA mutation can pass on without skipping a generation.

Who are BRCA1 or BRCA2 mutation carriers?

1. **Young women**. Notably, women with a BRCA1 mutation are typically diagnosed with breast cancer at a young age. Approximately half of breast cancers occur in BRCA1 mutation carriers before the age of 40. Breast cancer isn't just an old women's cancer.

2. **Both women and men**. BRCAs are not sex-linked genes. Hence, women are not the only BRCA mutation carriers. Men carry BRCA mutation too. People with a family history of cancer, particularly a known family history of BRCA1 or BRCA2 mutation, should be fully aware of being the potential carriers.

3. **Diverse race/ethnicity**. Americans can be BRCA mutation carriers, so can other populations worldwide. Breast cancer affects women of all race/ethnicity groups. However, black women have a higher prevalence of inherited mutations and die disproportionately from aggressive forms of the disease.[123]

What are the harmful effects of BRCA mutation?

For women with BRCA mutations, the lifetime risk of breast cancer is approximately 80 percent, and the chance of developing ovarian cancer is 54 percent.

Furthermore, BRCA mutations are also linked to other cancers.

- Women with a BRCA1 mutation are at risk for ovarian cancer and pancreatic cancer.
- Women with a BRCA2 mutation are at an increased risk for melanoma and pancreatic cancer.

- Other cancer risks include endometrial, skin and colon cancer.
- Men with BRCA2 mutation are at an increased risk of pancreatic cancer, prostate cancer, and melanoma.

Again, men can not only be potential carriers of BRCA gene mutations—and may pass on the mutation to their children—but also have a higher risk of developing other cancers.

Detecting a BRCA gene mutation—the pros and cons

First, you need to get a genetic counseling or check with an oncologist (or your physician) based on your own unique case so that you can make an informed decision.

You can get a genetic screening. Identifying or determining a BRCA gene mutation can be done with a blood test. Saliva can also be used for DNA mutation testing.

Genetic testing may spot unaffected yet high-risk individuals for prevention or closer monitoring. It can also help affected women or men choose the best proactive strategy or cancer therapy.

On the other hand, it's not a routine blood test for public screening. It's expensive, and it takes about a month to get the result.

Other practical ways to catch breast cancer early include the following:

1. Perform a self-examine of your breasts regularly. I cannot emphasize this basic practice enough because studies show that the majority of women with breast cancer found lumps in their breasts and brought to attention by themselves first.

2. Get a mammogram, and depending on the diagnosis, get an ultrasonography or MRI if necessary.
3. Recognize symptoms or early signs, and present them timely to get medical attention.
4. Consult your physicians, especially if you have a family history of breast cancer or any BRCA gene mutation.

What are common symptoms or early signs that you shouldn't ignore?

- Look for a lump in the breast. Sometimes it can be an area of lumpiness. You can find it through regular self-examination.
- The lump is not always painful or visible, but it can be felt.
- Is there any change in the skin around the nipple?
- Is there any unexpected nipple discharge or nipple retraction?
- Is there any change in the size or shape of the breast?
- Do you have any pain or discomfort in the area?
- Do you experience unexplained weight loss?
- There are signs that might indicate the cancer could be spreading. Do you feel a lump in the underarm area? Do you feel bone pain or other indications (e.g., shortness of breath, cough or unexplained gastrointestinal symptoms)?

Importantly, once you discover any symptoms, seek for medical consolation immediately and don't settle for any unclear evaluation. For instance, if you have a lump, even in the absence of pain, it's safe to have a biopsy and confirm its nature (i.e., cancerous or not).

In addition, you can educate others, enhance awareness, and

share accurate knowledge and screening techniques. All these help with early diagnosis and treatment of the disease.

Conclusion

Breast cancer is a major risk to women's health. It is such a scary, horrible, and challenging disease. BRCA gene mutations can lead to breast cancer and potentially other cancers. Early detection is the key to saving lives.

Undeniably, breast cancer prevention is for both women and men, and it is a year-round practice. Self-awareness is both essential and strategic. We cannot control our genes, but each of us can do something. Hence, act on self-care, i.e., stick to principles of early detection and stop heading toward unhealthy lifestyles, consequently reducing our cancer risk and preventing cancer.

Chapter 14 ─────────────────

Colon Cancer

The Best Way to Prevent Colon Cancer: Know Your Risk First

Colon (often referred to as colorectal) cancer remains the second leading cause of cancer deaths in the United States. It is the third most common cancer in both men and women, and around the world. Fortunately, colon cancer is preventable, especially when one adopts a healthy lifestyle.

With a rising incidence of colon cancer, the need for vigorous prevention and early detection is paramount.

To prevent colon cancer, one surefire step is to know the risk factors of colon cancer. For those who are unaware of or unclear about what the risks are, let's go through these factors.

Unmodifiable Risk Factors

Age

Colorectal cancer risk increases after age fifty. As you get older, your risk of colorectal cancer gets higher. Although more than 90 percent of the cases of this disease are diagnosed after age 55, more young adults are diagnosed with the disease, and the death rates from it are on the rise. That is why the ACS's updated screening guidelines in 2018 mainly recommend lowering the age to begin colorectal cancer screening at age 45 (i.e., five years younger than that previously) for adults at average risk.

Colon polyps

Polyps are small growth in the colon or rectum. Most of them are not cancerous, but some can become cancer, and they are commonly seen in people older than 50. A risk of colorectal cancer increases with the presence of polyps. Some polyps are inherited, such as those seen in familial adenomatous polyposis (FAP).

That explains why early detection by colon cancer screening is vitally important. A colonoscopy remains the gold standard for screening because it provides the best view of your entire colon, and cancerous polyps can also be removed during the procedure.

Family or personal history of cancer

Family history is significant. Having biologically close relatives (parents, brothers, sisters, or children) with colon cancer doubles an individual's risk of colon cancer. The lifetime risk of getting colon cancer for people with the inherited disorders increases measurably (e.g., 80 percent for Lynch syndrome and 100 percent for FAP).

Previous personal history of cancer or any inflammatory bowel disease increases the risk of colorectal cancer too.

Modifiable Risk Factors

Obesity

Obesity has been linked to a higher risk of various cancers, particularly an established risk factor for colorectal cancer. It will be addressed later in more detail.

Physical inactivity

Sedentary behavior or lifestyle increases a risk for many adverse health conditions such as diabetes, obesity, and cardiovascular disease. It can also increase the risk of several cancers, including colorectal cancer. So you may want to examine your TV-viewing time, internet-surfing time, and recreational and/or occupational sitting time.

Diet high in red meats but low in fiber

A diet high in red meats (e.g., beef, pork, lamb, or organ meat like liver) and processed meats (such as hot dogs and sausages) can increase colorectal cancer risk because of cancer-related chronic inflammation. Remember that processed red meats are known carcinogens. Refined flour and sugary drinks are also among the foods promoting inflammation.

On the other hand, a balanced diet that's heavy on fruits and vegetables and rich in fiber together with whole grains helps reduce inflammation, maintain a healthy weight, and protect your colon from cancerous growth.

Tobacco smoking

Tobacco smoking is a health hazard and one of the causes of cancer. It is certainly and causally linked to a higher risk for numerous types of cancer. Colorectal cancer is among them.

Heavy alcohol consumption

Excess alcohol intake causes cancer of several organs or tissues in the body, and indeed it plays a causative role in colorectal cancer. The fact is that heavy alcohol users tend to have low levels of folic acid in their bodies. Findings in humans indicate a clear link between colorectal cancer development and inadequate folate consumption. Folate deficiency may increase DNA damage through mechanisms that affect DNA repair genes.

Imbalanced gut bacteria

Emerging evidence has pointed to how bacteria may influence a risk of cancer. Millions of microbes in your gut interact with your immune system. Some are beneficial, but some are harmful. Experts believe that when bad bacteria attack your digestive system, you might suffer from inflammatory bowel diseases, and you are also at a higher risk for colorectal cancer because bad bacteria generate waste products that harm colon tissues and make them more vulnerable to malignancies.

Type 2 diabetes

Having type 2 diabetes increases a risk for colorectal cancer. Two diseases share some common risk factors. However, higher blood insulin and higher blood sugar with diabetes can cause inflammation in the colon, thereby facilitating the development of colorectal cancer. Having type 2 diabetes also tends to cast a less favorable prognosis after cancer diagnosis.

Please be aware that some of these risks are potentially enhanced in modern society. For example, TV watching is often associated with drinking sweetened beverages and eating junk foods. Sitting in your car during the long commute frequently comes with stress. Overall, these risk factors have a detrimental impact on colon cancer development.

Finally, it is paramount to underscore that only 5 to 6 percent of colon cancer is a result of inherited genetic mutations.[124] And having a family history doesn't automatically lead to altered genes implicated in the disease, because research indicates that there is a lack of the association between having a family history of colorectal cancer and genetic alterations in the tumors.[125] That means more than 90 percent of colon cancer incidents are attributed to gene mutations caused by diet, lifestyle, and environmental factors (e.g., carcinogenic effect or pollutant exposure, and/or infections)

I'll further elaborate on some strategies for preventing the development of colon cancer.

Early Detection—Recognize Early Signs and Go for Screenings

Two Critical Matters in Early Detection of Colorectal Cancer

According to the ACS, an estimated 135,430 cases of colorectal cancer will be diagnosed, and an estimated 50,260 deaths from the disease will occur in 2017 in the United States.

Within the predicted incidence, 71,420 will be men, and 64,010 will be women. Deaths will be 27,150 among men and 23,110 among women. Among cancer deaths, colon cancer is the second leading cause in men and the third leading cause in women among Americans.

These numbers make it clear that colorectal cancer affects both men and women, and dispels the myth that it is primarily a man's cancer.

Yet why are the statistics so large? Here are *two* areas many people often ignore or miss—a lack of adherence to the screening recommendation and a delay in presenting symptoms to a physician or oncologist.

Adherence to screening guidelines

Colonoscopies are recommended because they can help detect cancers at their earliest and most treatable stages. They can also detect precancerous polyps and remove them during the exam before they become cancerous.

Colonoscopy screening is a good example of how precision medicine impacts cancer prevention. Let me highlight the steps here.

First, there is a guideline to identify people at a risk for colon cancer and/or who need to be screened. Time for screening is recommended if you are 40 years old and have a family history or if you are 45 years old without a family history.

Second, the test can detect a growth (i.e., polyp) in the entire colon through imaging.

Finally, doctors can implement treatments immediately to prevent or slow down cancer progression (e.g., to surgically remove a benign growth or premalignant lesion during the screening or to start an aggressive therapy for a cancerous tumor).

If the result is normal, the colonoscopy should be repeated every 10 years up to the age of 75. If the test detects precancerous polyps, the physician will recommend repeating the exam more frequently.

Colonoscopy is a very effective and preferred screening method. As a result, colon cancer is highly preventable if caught in a precancerous stage. Studies demonstrate that this procedure can cut the odds of colon cancer death by approximately 50 percent.

Why should you go for a colonoscopy screening?

1. You gain significant value. Your anxiety, fear, or even feelings of embarrassment may be understandable. However, consider the following: Individuals undergo

this high-quality test under comfortable sedation, during which the entire colon and rectum are examined by a qualified gastroenterologist. Precancerous polyps can be found and removed safely. Can you see that this is a very valuable package of diagnosis and therapeutics for your colon health care?

2. You acquire rigorous clarity concerning your colon health. We want rigorous clarity in science, and surely, everyone wants thorough clarity when purchasing a house or insurance policy. It makes sense to seek rigorous clarity about a matter so critical to your health.

3. You benefit from one of the most effective cancer-prevention methods, and it is often covered by insurance.

Help your physician help you and how

In some cases, especially at an early stage, colon cancer may not present any symptoms. Again, that's why screening is vital to identify cancer early when prognosis and cure are optimistic.

Nevertheless, other folks may experience signs or symptoms such as

- blood in the stool;
- bleeding from the rectum;
- abdominal pain, cramping, or discomfort;
- feelings that the bowel isn't empty or bloating;
- changes in bowel habits (frequency, diarrhea, or constipation);
- difference in the stool (e.g., shape or color);
- unexplained fatigue or weakness; and/or
- unexplained weight loss.

That comes the point of early presentation. Don't dust off your doubts or warnings. Remember that nobody can read what's on your mind or what's going on in your life. If you don't visit or communicate with your doctor, it's likely he or she won't know about your cramps or unexplained changes in your bowel movements.

So devoting yourself to meeting screening guidelines is a key preventive measure, but another critical area is to counsel with your physician about possible warning signs.

Links between Obesity, Diabetes, and Colon Cancer

There are multiple causes of colon cancer. They include cellular, molecular, and genetic factors as well as dietary and lifestyle factors. Here I'm going to focus on one significant yet modifiable risk factor—obesity.

A glimpse at the numbers

The incidence rate of obesity is alarmingly high among US adults based on the CDC data. The obesity rates among different age groups include the following: middle-aged (40.2 percent), older (37.0 percent), and younger (32.3 percent). Also, about 17 percent of children and adolescents (age two through nineteen) are obese.

More than 30 million people in the United States have diabetes. More than 84 million Americans have prediabetes, a condition that can lead to type 2 diabetes. Note that an estimated one in two seniors has prediabetes.

Obesity may be a factor in approximately 300,000 deaths each year. Diabetes caused 83,564 deaths in 2017, and colorectal cancer caused more than 50,000 deaths in 2018.

A look beyond the numbers

Obesity is a leading cause of diabetes, a disease for which the body fails to control blood sugar levels. High blood sugar levels are characteristic of both obesity and diabetes. What is less well known is that diabetes and obesity are also linked to an increase in cancer risk.

In fact, obesity contributes to many types of cancer (colon, esophageal, thyroid, breast, prostate, uterine, kidney, pancreas, gallbladder, and non-Hodgkin lymphoma) and it's also linked to heart disease, stroke, and other chronic illnesses.

Convincing evidence shows that obesity and diabetes are associated with an increased risk of developing colon cancer.

Intrinsic links between obesity, diabetes, and colon cancer are vastly complicated. One clear tie is sugar. High blood sugar also makes us predisposed to cancer by increasing the activity of a gene involved in cancer progression. Apparently, dietary sugar is a link tying together obesity, diabetes, and colon cancer, and thus, excess sugar intake has an impact on our risk for cancer.

Certainly, other links play a causal role. Chronic inflammation is a central process that likely leads obese individuals to an elevated risk of diabetes and colon cancer. In fact, all three conditions also share a common inflammatory path involving multiple inflammation-promoting factors or biomarkers and nuclear factors.

An important outlook and strategy

Both obesity and diabetes can be prevented through lifestyle modification—balanced diet, physical activity, and weight management among other measures. Interventions at multiple levels, including individuals, health care systems, and communities, should be proactive in order to optimize the colon health.

How Fiber Protects You against Colon Cancer

Because fiber-rich diets can protect you from colon cancer, I'd like to help you understand why fiber could be your secret weapon in fighting colon cancer based on some new research evidence.

As outlined in this schematic illustration, GPR109A (a receptor termed G-protein-coupled receptor 109A, i.e., the lock in the picture) can help fight colon cancer.[126, 127] It is located on the colon epithelial cells—the cells covering the surface of your gastrointestinal tract. But how does GPR109A carry out the mission?

Schematic Illustration 5. How dietary fibers help prevent colon cancer.

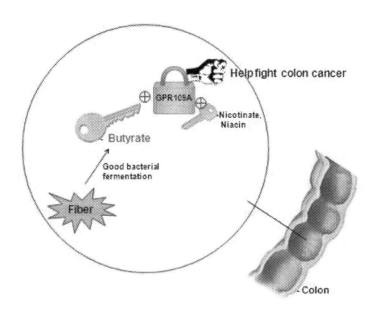

First, the receptor GPR109A is a tumor suppressor, which means it protects a cell from its progression to cancer. But it cannot operate alone. Just think about how a lock and a key work together. For a receptor (like a lock) to perform any function, it needs the binding of a ligand (a molecule, which functions as a key) to form a biochemical complex. The interaction subsequently initiates certain cellular change.

What is the ligand (the key) for GPR109A (the lock)? In this case, they are two keys—niacin (vitamin B3) and butyrate, a by-product from bacteria fermentation of dietary fiber. Under physiological conditions, niacin is not present at a concentration high enough to activate the receptor, though it is a normal biological component in the blood and cells. On the other hand, butyrate is the physiological ligand (the key) for GPR109A in the colon.

Thus, butyrate is more relevant and important in fighting colon cancer.

When butyrate binds to GPR109A, the activation of GPR190A triggers a signaling pathway that can set off the immune cells in the colon to produce anti-inflammatory molecules. As a result, it has anti-inflammation and antitumor effects.

Again, the good news is that these events take place only in the colon!

This powerful knowledge provides one lifesaving reason that fiber-rich foods promote colon health. Based on overwhelming evidence, a higher intake of vegetables has been associated with a lower risk of colon cancer. Heavy consumption of plant-based foods has also been associated with a reduced risk of colon cancer.

Inadequate fiber intake can cause a low level of butyrate and consequently promote inflammation in the gut. To have a sufficient supply of butyrate and a healthy colon, it's essential to consume plenty of fiber-rich foods such as fruits, vegetables, and whole grains.

In brief, butyrate-activated GPR109A collaboration can suppress chronic inflammation and support colon cancer prevention. Because butyrate is derived from fiber digestion made by good bacteria in the gut, you need abundant fiber-rich, plant-based foods to ward off colon cancer.

Chapter 15 ———————————

Childhood Cancer

How to Prevent Childhood Cancer

Your cute baby girl is the joy of your life, yet she is suffering from leukemia. A neighbor's little boy with a gorgeous smile just completed his cancer treatment. Sadly, many precious young lives have been taken away by childhood cancers.

Approximately 15,700 children are diagnosed with cancer each year. Among them, an estimated 1,960 deaths are expected. Childhood cancer remains the leading cause of death in children (younger than fifteen years old). Are you aware of these sober statistics?

Sadly and alarmingly, there is an increase in childhood cancer incidences worldwide.

Losing a child to cancer is an unthinkable pain and despair to all parents, which is why we should call to prevent the worst loss and why I emphasize education and empowerment, particularly on potential risk factors and powerful strategic actions to prevent childhood cancer.

Let's dive right into it.

Characteristics of childhood cancers

The types of cancer that develop in children and adolescents vastly differ from those occurring in adults. As observed, cancers of the lung, colon, breast, prostate, and skin strike most adults domestically and globally.

Conversely, the most common types of childhood cancer are leukemia, tumors of the brain and central nervous system, and lymphoma. Some cancers from embryonic cells and/or in developing organs include neuroblastoma (peripheral nervous system), medulloblastoma (brain), nephroblastoma or Wilms tumor (kidney), and retinoblastoma (retina of the eye), which are rarely seen in adults. Also, incidences of these cancers vary by children's age.

What exactly causes childhood cancer remains unclear. Different cancers have different risk factors. Again, unlike many adult cancers, lifestyle-related risk factors (e.g., tobacco smoking, alcohol consumption, physical inactivity and poor diet, etc.) do not play a significant role in a child's risk of developing cancer. On the other hand, most childhood cancers result from an inherited gene mutation or environmental factors or both.

Am I suggesting that we cannot do anything to prevent childhood cancer? No, I am not.

Children are our treasure, and children's health is our nation's wealth. I'll proceed to prevention with knowledge and more effective approaches later.

Eight aspects of childhood cancer's unique challenges

Although remarkable progress has been made in advance of innovative or healing therapies, childhood cancers create unique challenges for us, for kids, and for their families. It is of considerable importance to know *why* from the following eight aspects:

1. The common cancers that develop in children and adolescents differ from those that occur in adults (as mentioned previously).
2. Cancers in children and adolescents vary among ages. And each age group needs its own target treatment and care.
3. Young kids are still in their developmental stages and vulnerable to cancer treatments. For instance, treatment like radiation can harm their organs and tissues.
4. Lifestyle-related risk factors play little role in childhood cancers, unlike those seen in many cancers of adults. However, other external risk factors—such as infectious agents and environmental pollutants—have been linked to childhood cancers. Radiation exposure might be unavoidable because of the need for cancer treatment.
5. Prevention is challenging too. Pediatric cancers are generally caused by some key genetic mutations or changes. However, prevention is better than cure, and there are rooms for it.
6. Childhood cancers are rare, complex, and aggressive in nature and in a small population, thereby posing challenges to the research and discovery of new therapies (one of them being the limited number of clinical trials conducted).
7. Because of the biological heterogeneity within specific subtypes of certain cancer, each childhood cancer requires its own set of treatments. Although some cancers that are seemingly different can be treated alike, the one-size-fits-all approach is not an effective one.

8. Survivors of childhood cancer face a lifelong risk of developing secondary cancers. First, the treatments themselves have the potential to cause cancer. Second, young survivors also have to live with late adverse health problems for the rest of their lives.

While we're embracing the heartbreak of childhood cancers, it is important to identify the survival challenges and needs, because sometimes the late effect from childhood cancer treatment can seriously affect one's body and mind. We should improve the quality of life for young cancer patients and their families.

Unique Risk Factors

Children are not small adults. In general, their care challenges are attributed to multiple factors, including their growth and development, psychological features, health condition, socioeconomic status, family and cultural dynamics, nurture at home, and support outside of the home.

Childhood cancers are full of complexity and unknown variables. However, some risk factors for childhood cancer have been established.

Genetic or inherent risk factors include parental age, birth weight, and congenital abnormalities. Some pediatric cancer incidences also vary by age, sex, and race or ethnicity. Non-genetic risk factors are controllable and preventable, and these include the following:

- high doses of radiation (The human fetus is very sensitive to radiation.);
- RF radiation;
- exposure to environmental carcinogens, pesticides, and air pollution;

- exposure to infections;
- prior chemotherapy; and
- prenatal and perinatal lifestyle factors.

Note that radiation is a known carcinogen, although medically applied radiation is unescapable in cancer treatment. Meanwhile, be aware of nonionizing radiation, particularly extremely low-frequency electromagnetic fields (EMFs). The IARC has classified RF radiation as a possible human carcinogen [Group 2B]. Growing evidence indicates that mobile phone related EMFs is an attributable factor to brain tumors, particularly because of the thinner skulls, still developing nervous system and undeveloped brain in young children.[128, 129] Brain tumors are one of the leading causes of cancer death in children.

It is also worth stressing the role of prenatal and perinatal lifestyle factors in childhood cancer development. Issues such as nutritional deficiency, maternal smoking, alcohol consumption or substance abuse, and certain maternal medications all make babies vulnerable to adverse environmental exposure. Then more frequency of timing, longer duration, more quantity and intensity of adverse exposure can have a greater impact on epigenetic change, early development and cancer risk accumulation during life. Nevertheless, socioeconomic inequalities are also associated with risk for cancer, other non-communicable diseases and premature death.

Childhood Leukemia

Childhood leukemia is the most common pediatric cancer worldwide, embodying one-third of all cancers that occur in children under 15 years old. It is the leading cause of cancer deaths in children. Therefore, I elaborate in more details on the role of various risk factors in this disease.

Leukemia is an aberrant hyper-proliferation of immature blood cells, which does not form a solid tumor mass. There are four main subgroups of leukemia—acute lymphocytic leukemia (ALL), acute myeloid leukemia (AML), chronic lymphocytic leukemia (CLL), and chronic myeloid leukemia (CML). ALL and AML are the most common malignancies of children.

Leukemia risk factors can be classified as noncontrollable and controllable ones.[130]

Noncontrollable risk factors include

- gender (because more incidences occur in male children);
- age (depending on the subtype of leukemia);
- blood disorders;
- congenital syndromes (e.g., Down's syndrome):
- genetic susceptibility; and
- family history (though with only certain leukemias, specifically CLL).

Controllable risk factors include the following:

- **Parental exposure**

  Because of the young age at diagnosis and compelling evidence that many affected children bear chromosomal damages before birth, various parental factors are involved in the diseases, including

  a) maternal factors during pregnancy, such as smoking, fetal loss, and stillbirth, all of which are significantly linked to leukemia;
  b) maternal infections during pregnancy (thus increasing the risk of leukemia);

  c) paternal or maternal occupational exposure to pesticides (e.g., agricultural workers);

  d) parental use of alcohol; and

  e) parental usage of illicit drugs or controlled substances.

- **Viral infections**

Viral infections may be responsible for genetic changes in the development of childhood leukemia despite a lower rate of incidence (approximately 10 percent). The viruses with high prevalence involve Epstein-Barr virus, human T-lymphotropic retrovirus, human herpes virus type 6 or 8, human parvovirus B19, and H. pylori.

 The exposures to common infections in utero, during prenatal or postnatal period and early life contribute to the etiology of childhood leukemia through various transmittable pathways.

- **Radiations**

This includes high doses of ionizing radiation or radon (radioactive gas), especially for ALL, AML. The exposure to nonionizing EMFs is also linked to the risk of childhood leukemia though further studies are needed.

- **Environmental pollution**

Environmental factors include occupational or individual exposure to benzene, pesticides, indoor and outdoor air pollution. They are reminiscent of some distinct incident patterns by sex, age and geography. Environmental factors can influence the genetic predisposition and thus plays a role in initiating leukemia. Noticeably, benzene and ionizing radiation are two environmental exposures strongly associated with the development of childhood AML and ALL.[130]

- **Smoking**

   Tobacco smoke, active or passive exposure, is the foremost cause of preventable morbidity and mortality in the world. More critically, when the exposure starts prenatally (i.e., passive exposure from the placenta to the fetus), it can lead to not only negative health outcomes, but also experimental or regular smoking and ultimately habitual smoking or addiction.

- **Previous cancer treatments**

   Children have a greater chance of developing leukemia if they have undergone previous chemotherapy or radiation therapy for other types of cancer.

Cancer is a significant cause of death in children and adolescents despite its relatively rare prevalence before the age of 20 years. Knowing the unique challenges and risk factors of childhood cancer, are you determined to be a part of the fighting force? If so, here are some actions you can take.

How to Prevent Childhood Cancers

The best strategy is primary prevention—to reduce the exposure to known cancer risk factors affecting children. This commitment has proven effective. At the same time, you can ensure secondary prevention with early detection.

Keeping cancer risk factors in mind, each of us can do our

part at each stage of a child's life, particularly commit to the following actions.

1. **Start from preconception, and take good care of yourself throughout the pregnancy period.**

   - Consume adequate nutrition. Strong evidence suggests that the vitamin intake and nutrient status from maternal preconception to perinatal period influence the cancer risk of the infant or child.
   - Avoid or minimize your exposure to secondhand and thirdhand smoke.
   - Refrain from an unhealthy diet, tobacco, alcohol or substance use, unnecessary medications, and radiation (i.e., any causal link to childhood cancer).

2. **Detect cancer early by genetic consultation and testing.**

   DNA makes up our genes and certainly influences our risks for developing certain diseases, including cancer. A child may inherit DNA mutations from a parent, and that can increase his or her risk of cancer. The alterations can be present in every cell of the child's body, and the mutation can be identified by testing the DNA of blood cells or other cells in the body.

   Genetic consulting is also constructive for someone with a history of familial cancers or having an uncertainty of genetic abnormality. The consultation can help evaluate how parents' occupational, environmental, medical or other exposures may contribute to a child's cancer risk.

3. **Stop smoking**, **especially during pregnancy**.

Children deserve a smoke-free world.

A cigarette releases more than seven thousand chemicals, seventy of those are known carcinogens. Tobacco products damage almost every organ in the body, including the mouth, eyes, lungs, guts, reproductive organs, bladder, and bones.

4. **Eliminate or minimize exposure to toxins and carcinogens in daily life**

I understand that it's virtually impossible to escape environmental pollutants and toxic chemicals entirely in modern society—at home or from environment at large. Environmental pollutants or toxins are probably the most invasive and cumulative hazard during a child's early development, and of course, they pose a threat to a child's health.

Of significant concern is that children are at a higher risk of acute and chronic exposure to environmental contaminants. Children are more vulnerable because they absorb more than adults exposed to pollutants at equal levels.

Endless exposure to toxic chemicals through air, water, foods, and everyday products results in a serious impact on public health too. It's critical to underscore that only a small number of chemical exposures are known, yes, there are many unknown or unidentified ones.

That's why environmental protection is vitally important, and a green planet signifies healthful generations. Unquestionably, you can make every effort and conscious choices to avoid your exposure to the everyday toxins or hidden carcinogens.

5. Grow your own toxin-free vegetables, or buy organic.

In this way, you will get more vitamins, more minerals, and more micronutrients. You will also eat pesticides-free food. Plus, gardening helps you stay physically active.

6. Delay the time your kids use cell phones or other mobile devices.

Take preventive measures on the exposure to RF radiation associated with mobile phones. At least delay the time they start using them, and limit the time they use them. It's wise to monitor and control kids' screen time for their safety and quality of sleep as well.

7. Foster individual hygiene and infection prevention.

Because of the role that bacterial or viral infections play in the origin of cancer, it's essential to teach your children good hygiene habits.

8. Get vaccinated.

Vaccinations save lives. Parents should encourage and educate their children or teens to get vaccinated against HPV and practice safe sex. Health care providers should also advise and educate youth.

It's important that you adhere to the recommended childhood immunizations. Don't allow any unfounded or misguided fear about vaccines to influence you and pressure you to make a dangerous decision.

9. **Identify a critical window of susceptibility and prevention among youth**.

Pay close attention to preadolescents, adolescents, and young adults. Early life exposures during times of rapid growth and development may impact one's later life. And there are also unique psychosocial needs of this age group.

10. **Cultivate and live a healthy lifestyle.**

One important approach in fighting childhood cancers— and all cancer—is for parents to model and cultivate a healthy lifestyle for their children at an early age. Then they can pass the *baton* to the next generation so that they can lower their children's risk of getting cancer later in life.

Lifestyle factors usually take years or decades to influence cancer risk, but it's never too late to develop a healthy lifestyle. Nevertheless, parental lifestyle factors play a crucial role in a child's health outcome.

Eat plenty of nutrient-rich and antioxidant-rich foods, engage in physical activities, maintain a healthy weight, and keep a positive attitude. Ensure your overall well-being by getting enough sleep and practicing sun protection.

The earlier children adopt a healthy lifestyle, the better off they will be in their overall health, and the more likely they will stay with healthful living in the long run. Living a healthy lifestyle can benefit not only yourself and your children's health but also the future generations to come. Early adopted healthy habits likely make it easier for your children to take the baton and run the next laps to their bright destinies.

11. Improve care and support for pediatric cancer patients and survivors (including all generations because some are adults now).

The ever-increasing number of childhood cancer survivors (as many as two-thirds) is creating public health issues as they transfer or progress into adulthood. Consider what their lives after cancer look like, particularly their painful and practical challenges in daily life. There may be overlooked care issues such as long-term effects due to previous cancer treatment, reduced or discontinued follow-up with their pediatric oncologists, and awareness level from adult health care providers of survivors' health risks, etc.

In addition, children who survive their initial cancers remain at risk for having cancer recurrence or developing new cancers (secondary malignancies), yet a majority of cancer survivors do not receive risk-based care.

12. Team up and receive care from society.

You can receive help in a school and/or community setting. Family dynamics, socioeconomic status or poverty level and issues of violence can all contribute to pediatric health challenges.

Furthermore, advocate health care models or payment changes because these tactics can ease the financial burdens of childhood cancer treatment and encourage disease prevention.

Summary

Cancer impacts our children's well-being and lives. We all have the responsibility to take care of children and protect them from a variety of dangers, including interruptions during pregnancy, genetic abnormalities, perinatal injuries, congenital defects, malnutrition, environmental hazards, infections, poverty, violence, and trauma. We can do a lot to help address their unique needs and find solutions when we open our hearts and minds.

Chapter 16 ———————————————

Leukemia

Leukemia Risk and Preventable Factors

Leukemia is a group of malignant disorders of the blood and bone marrow. What causes leukemia is not entirely known, but established risk factors for leukemia can be categorized as follows:

Genetic and familial

The striking difference between childhood leukemia and adult leukemia lies in their genetics. In childhood leukemia structure alterations of genes are more common than genetic mutations while the opposite is seen in adult leukemia. There are genetic damages in childhood leukemia too. And there is age-associated variation in disease incidence. Particularly, AML is much less common in young children but more prevalent with age (less than 10 percent in children younger than two years of age and 40 percent in adults).

In addition, children with leukemia are born with genetic mutations, whereas genetic mutations in adults are more due to accumulated environmental effects on genes over time, which might also explain why leukemia is typically seen in older adults (i.e., at their sixties to eighties).

Environmental

Environmental factors such as benzene, high doses of ionizing radiation, EMFs, and chemotherapy play a role.

Benzene is a proven risk factor and a known carcinogen. Occupational exposure to benzene increases the risk of leukemia in a dose-dependent pattern. Other sources of benzene exposure can come from cigarette smoke, car exhaust, industrial emissions, building materials, paints, and adhesives.

Medically applied radiation and chemotherapy are also clearly associated with subsequent development of leukemia.

EMF-related radiation can exist in daily life (e.g., microwave, TV, computer, etc.). The EPA recommends a safe exposure of 0.5 mG to 205 mG (i.e., milliGauss used to measure EMFs). For example, when you are one meter or three feet away from a microwave oven, your exposure is up to 25 mG.

The role of other environmental factors such as indoor and outdoor pollution is uncertain and requires more studies.

Lifestyle

While benzene, radiation, and chemotherapy are more attributable risk factors, lifestyle factors such as smoking, obesity, and exposure to EMF show weak associations with leukemia.

So prevention of this disease is certainly possible by avoiding the exposure to the outlined risk factors and the unsafe behaviors linked to leukemia.

Eight Things You Can Do to Avoid or Minimize Benzene Exposure

Is benzene present in your workplace, community, or home?

Benzene is a widely used chemical. It is a colorless, flammable, and volatile organic compound with a pleasant, sweet smell. Benzene is produced by the combustion of crude oil and gasoline. It is found in nature (e.g., in volcanoes and forest fires) and in cigarette smoke. It is also used to manufacture many types of products such as

- plastics,
- resins,
- nylon and synthetic fibers,
- rubbers,
- lubricants,
- dyes,
- detergents,
- drugs, and
- pesticides.

Benzene is a known carcinogen [Group 1] and a common environmental pollutant that has been linked to leukemia.[20, 131] Benzene exposure can also lead to numerous noncancerous health problems that affect normal functions of the vital systems in the body such as the cardiovascular, nervous, immune, endocrine, and reproductive systems.

But how do you protect yourself and your family from any health hazards resulting from excessive benzene exposure? Here are eight actions you can take:

1. Get well informed. Know where benzene is in your vicinity, including what home products contain benzene.
2. Avoid tobacco smoke, including passive smoke. Benzene is one of the carcinogens released from tobacco smoke. It is estimated that about half of benzene exposure in the United States is from cigarette smoking.

3. Reduce outdoor exposure in areas around gas stations and areas surrounding motor vehicle exhaust or industrial emissions, where the air contains higher levels of benzene.

4. Keep indoor environments ventilated. Benzene in indoor air comes from products like glues, paints, furniture wax, detergents, and certain drugs. According to the CDC, indoor air generally contains higher levels of benzene than outdoor air.[132]

5. Read labels when you shop for groceries, especially when buying soft drinks. Some ingredients (e.g., benzoates and vitamin C) in many beverages can form this carcinogen and heat may speed up the process though its levels are relatively low.

6. Know your workplace exposure and protect yourself properly. Since people working in industries that make or use benzene may vulnerably be open to high levels of it, make sure that your company takes preventive measures and you wear safety gear (e.g., clothing, goggles, etc.).

7. Become aware of other environmental sources of benzene. For instance, benzene can leak from underground storage tanks or from hazardous waste sites. Waste sites containing benzene can contaminate well water.

8. If you consider that you've experienced any overexposure to benzene, consult your doctor and get tested for a level of benzene exposure.

Overall, health consequences associated with benzene exposure are serious, so don't overlook this dangerous substance. For your safety and wellness, take preventive measures.

Chapter 17 ──────────────

Lung Cancer

Three Key Sources of Lung Cancer Development

When I think about lung cancer, I replay horrifying memories of my dad being cruelly taken away by this disease within a month after diagnosis and my mother-in-law being painfully tortured for two years after her lung cancer surgery. And they both were nonsmokers.

Lung cancer is the leading cause of cancer deaths among both men and women in the United States and worldwide. You may have a story to tell too.

Paradoxically, lung cancer is one of the most preventable types of cancer. Because smoking is the killer in approximately 90 percent of men and 80 percent of women who have died of lung cancer, the most effective prevention and measures are cessation of cigarette smoking and elimination of tobacco exposure.

Here, aside from genetic factors and preexisting lung diseases, I'm focusing on three important factors.

1. Tobacco smoking and passive exposure

Cigarette smoking is an indisputable risk factor for lung cancer. Much has been done by quit smoking campaigns. Yet stores still sell cigarettes, and folks still buy and smoke them. Let's make this message clear: Smoking destroys your key weapon to fight cancer!

Why? Tobacco smoking causes a profound mutation of genes, especially the mutation of a tumor suppressor called TP53, the gene that helps you fight cancer! Fascinatingly, TP53 is also referred to as the *guardian of the genome*.[133] Research findings demonstrate that elephants (Asian and Africa) have 20 copies of the tumor suppressor gene TP53, while humans have only one copy per set of chromosomes, which may explain why the cancer rate is significantly lower in elephants than it is in humans.[134] Why would anyone destroy this powerful anticancer weapon? And remember that exposure to secondhand smoke can also lead to dire consequences.

2. Dietary or food carcinogenic factors

Diet is also an etiologic factor in developing lung cancer because this occurs through the ingestion of food mutagens.[135-137] Food mutagens or carcinogens tend to aim at specific organs rather than affecting every organ in the body. Specifically, *N*-nitrosamines and PAH target lung and gastrointestinal tract.

Food quality and sources are of major concern. You may have no idea what's hidden inside your food. Three common factors should be highlighted because they can potentially cause lung and other cancers:

Improper cooking

Meat (beef, pork, fish, or poultry) cooked at high temperatures generates cancer-causing compounds such as HCAs and PAHs. In many studies, rodents fed a diet containing HCAs developed lung cancer and cancers of the breast, colon, liver, skin, and prostate. PAHs promote cancers of the lung and gastrointestinal tract as well as leukemia. Analysis of human urinary samples confirmed the result from mutagenic exposure to high-heat cooked meat.

Processed foods

The WHO and IARC have classified processed meat as a human carcinogen, and processed red meats (especially done by curing, smoking, salting or adding chemical preservatives) play a role in carcinogenesis. Food additives and/or coloring substances such as nitrite and nitrate are considered mutagens. They trigger mutation, and then accumulated mutations may initiate or proceed to cancer.

Junk foods

Other dietary factors include the overindulgence of sugar, fat, sodium, and total calories. These factors lead to fat buildup, obesity, and potentially genetic alteration, all of which promote cancer.

3. Environmental carcinogens and Air pollution

Because most lung cancer cases result from inhaling carcinogens, it's also critical to stay away from environmental hazards that are risk factors for lung cancer. These include

- radon,
- asbestos,
- air pollution,
- certain occupational materials (coal, tar, arsenic, nickel, chromium, and cement dust),

- radiation, and
- products with toxic chemicals.

Lung cancer is largely preventable by eliminating tobacco smoke and avoiding radon exposure. Radon, a colorless, odorless and naturally occurring radioactive gas, is a known human carcinogen. It causes approximately 21,000 deaths from lung cancer annually, making it the second most crucial cause of lung cancer after smoking.

Radon and its decayed products can be found in all rocks and soil, even in water sometimes. It may also be found in indoor environments such as homes, workplaces, and schools. Radon can easily leak from the ground into the air and decay. When breathing in, the particles can damage DNA, and potentially cause lung diseases or lung cancer.

It's worth noting that the populations—particularly among individuals younger than 30 and those who are non- or less-educated—don't know what radon is. Of adults who heard about radon, the majority of them don't know that radon causes lung cancer. Nevertheless, radon testing rates were also low.[138] Certainly, some confusion with carbon monoxide exists too. It's of importance to know that household carbon monoxide detectors (fire alarms) do not detect radon.

Putting it all together, a modern lifestyle of convenience is often mixed with outdoor air pollution by environmental toxins and indoor air pollution because of smoking or VOCs along with food contaminants and carcinogens.

Quite disturbing and concerning, isn't it?

Ladies, you should especially watch out because women are at a higher risk of developing lung cancer than men, whether you smoke or not!

Occupational Chemicals Linked to Lung Cancer

Everyday exposure in the workplace is a serious concern because the exposure to harmful substances at high levels and over a long period of time can be a lethal threat to your health. It's essential to understand what common occupational substances may increase your risk of lung cancer and how you can protect yourself.

How to raise your awareness

The IARC has identified several occupational materials/agents as lung carcinogens or possible carcinogens to humans. Numerous studies have established a causative link between overexposure to common occupational materials and an increased risk of lung cancer.[20]

Occupational and/or environmental substances associated with lung cancer include

- asbestos,
- aluminum,
- arsenic,
- chromium,
- formaldehyde,
- nickel,
- silica,
- coal gasification,
- coal tar,
- soot,
- diesel fumes, and
- radon, radiation.

For the general population, although the exposure levels to

most of these agents are likely insufficient to produce serious health damage, it is wise to become informed and cautious.

How to protect yourself from potential lung carcinogens

Here are ten tips for your benefit.

1. Keep informed, especially know what you are exposed to in the workplace and what you can do to safeguard yourself.
2. Always wear protective clothing, items, and equipment as occupational safety requires.
3. Read the labels and follow the instructions. This is extremely necessary whenever and wherever you handle chemical-containing products.
4. Stick to the rules or regulations on dealing with hazard wastes.
5. Make sure that your employer is aware of certain job-related potential danger to human health, and always have protective measurements in place.
6. Take your shoes off at the door to avoid tracking potential toxins from the bottom of the shoes around your home.
7. Separate your work clothing from those you wear off-work or items of your family when you're doing laundry, if necessary.
8. Become mindful and take precautions about the chemicals you use in your home.
9. Check radon levels in your house. The EPA defines *high exposure* to radon as its level being 4 pCi/L and above.
10. Avoid or minimize unnecessary radiation exposure.

These practices are particularly imperative to people who are already at risk for lung cancer, including but not limited to those

- with previous lung diseases such as tuberculosis and chlamydia pneumonia,
- with a family history of lung cancer,
- with compromised immunity, and
- who are smokers and secondhand (or passive) smokers.

Remember that early detection is key. If you experience any symptoms such as frequent cough, coughing out blood, breathing difficulty, wheezing, chest pain, or unexplained weight loss, consult your doctor.

In contrast to advances in the screening of breast, prostate, and colon cancer, progress with the early detection of lung cancer is falling behind.

A brief update on lung cancer screening

Patients with lung cancer are often symptomless yet have a poor prognosis. There is no well-accepted routine for lung cancer screening currently, and lung cancer is diagnosed mainly by chest x-rays (which are less effective at an early stage and less costly) and CT (which is significantly more sensitive than chest x-rays for identifying lung cancer when it's small and asymptomatic). CT scans, however, are expansive and not feasible for large population screening. Because of its sensitivity, abnormalities revealed by CT scans are not all cancerous.

Other tests and promising methods include (but are not limited to)

1) sputum cytology, which is used to check mucus brought up from the lungs by coughing;

2) biopsy for area(s) of abnormality, which is effective though risky;

3) lung cancer biomarkers show promises yet need careful validation (bearing in mind that although numerous biomarkers for lung cancer have been studied, their specificity and sensitivity are unsatisfactory clinically); and

4) autofluorescence bronchoscopy, which is used to help detect mucosal changes of early lesions that may appear subtle on normal bronchoscopy.

Advances in lung cancer screening are still underway and combined testing approaches can support a clinical diagnosis. After all, early detection is a lifesaving decision and measure, particularly for people at a higher risk.

Chapter 18 ——————————

Pancreatic Cancer

Emerging Evidence on Pancreatic Cancer Risks

Pancreatic cancer is a highly lethal malignancy and still has an extremely poor prognosis or outcome with an overall survival of 5 percent over five years.

This is a keynote topic because of the striking statistics of growing incidence and mortality of pancreatic cancer. In 2017, estimated 53,670 people would be diagnosed with pancreatic cancer, and more than 43,000 deaths would occur from this disease in the United States alone. Then there were approximately 55,440 new cases and 44,330 deaths in 2018, according to the ACS.

Looking at the trend, pancreatic cancer's incidences and deaths have been rising in recent decades, and it is expected to become the second leading cause of cancer-related death in the United States by 2030.[139]

Pancreatic cancer is remarkably aggressive. However, because of ambiguous symptoms or even a lack of symptoms, not to mention the lack of an effective screening method, it's rarely diagnosed at an early stage, which means leaving no opportunity for surgical intervention. Moreover, the disease is difficult to treat because of its resistance to radiotherapy and chemotherapy. Thus, the disease's cruelty creates a tremendous emotional burden for both patients and their loved ones. Even for survivors, the battles and treatments are brutal.

This doesn't mean we can't do anything.

To treat this devastating disease early and save more lives, it is crucial to identify risk factors of pancreatic cancer and target high-risk individuals for effective screening. A better understanding of associated risk factors for pancreatic cancer can pinpoint preventive strategies to reduce its incidence. Therefore, steps to help prevent pancreatic cancer need everybody's attention.

Here I've compiled a list of risk factors for pancreatic cancer from a wealth of evidence over the past decades.

Established risk factors

1. **Cigarette smoking:** It is consistently associated with a twofold increase in pancreatic cancer risk. Carcinogens in tobacco products cause DNA damage, which leads to abnormal cell growth.

2. **Excessive alcohol:** Heavy alcohol consumption is linked to chronic pancreatitis—a known risk factor for pancreatic cancer. This is because during metabolism of alcohol in humans, carcinogenic acetaldehyde and fatty acid ethyl esters cause pancreatitis-like injury.

3. **Obesity:** Obesity produces an inflammatory state. Visceral obesity (belly fat) is linked to an increased risk for pancreatic and other cancers, independent of general obesity measured by BMI.

4. **Chronic inflammatory conditions:** Chronic pancreatitis is clearly a strong risk factor for pancreatic cancer. Liver cirrhosis (i.e., scarring of the liver from hepatitis and heavy alcohol consumption) is also a risk factor.

5. **Diabetes:** Type 2 diabetes is among a cluster of metabolic syndromes that include hypertension, dyslipidemia, insulin resistance, and obesity.

6. **Age:** The risk of developing pancreatic cancer increases with age. Most people are diagnosed after age 65. (The cancer almost always strikes after age 45, and 71 is the average age at diagnosis).

7. **Gender:** Men are more likely to develop pancreatic cancer.

8. **Family history of pancreatic cancer or certain cancer:** A family history of ovarian, breast, and colorectal cancers could also be associated with an increased risk for pancreatic cancer.[140]

9. **Inherited genetic mutation or syndromes:** Genetic factors account for approximately 10 percent of pancreatic cancer cases. These conditions include BRCA2 gene mutation, hereditary breast-ovarian cancer (HBOC) syndrome, hereditary pancreatitis, Lynch syndrome, and familial atypical mole-malignant melanoma syndrome (FAMMM).

Emerging risk factors

1. **Environmental risk:** Exposure to mutagenic nitrosamines, organ-chlorinated compounds or heavy metals is involved in the initiating phase of pancreatic cancer. Accumulated asbestos fibers may play a role in the progression of the disease.[141]

2. **Gut microbiota:** These bacteria are invisible, but don't overlook them. The role of the microbiota in the development of pancreatic diseases is increasingly accepted.[142, 143] Gut bacteria translocation and small intestine bacterial overgrowth have been found in acute pancreatitis and chronic pancreatitis respectively.

Imbalance of gut microbiota is also related to other risk factors for pancreatic cancer (such as smoking, diabetes, and obesity).

3. **Infection:** Pancreatic cancer may also be attributed to Helicobacter pylori (*H. pylori*) infection or a pathogen for periodontal disease (named *porphyromonas gingivalis*).[143-145] Furthermore, oral dysbiosis may increase a risk of developing pancreatic cancer.

4. **Ionizing radiation:** Most relevant evidence for this link comes from studies done on workers who have had occupational exposure.

Preventable or modifiable risk factors

1. **Smoking:** Smoking is the biggest preventable cause of cancer.

2. **Obesity, especially abdominal adiposity:** Obesity is a significant risk factor for more than ten types of cancer, severe morbidities, and premature death. It is also a major modifiable risk factor for these chronic diseases. Heavy fat around the belly area is alarmingly harmful. Research suggests that the larger a waist circumference, the higher a risk for pancreatic cancer.[146]

3. **Type 2 diabetes:** Lifestyle modification and weight management can prevent or delay diabetes. See more detail in the coming segment below.

4. **Sedentary behavior:** Physical inactivity is directly and independently linked to multiple types of cancer and obesity.

5. **Alcohol consumption:** It raises the risk for several types of cancer. And alcohol can fan the flames of diabetes complications.

6. **Dietary factors:** A diet high in red and processed meats, fat, calories, and fructose may increase cancer

risk. In contrast, a diet rich in whole grains, fiber, vegetables and fruits is associated with reduced cancer risk.

7. **Chronic inflammation:** Anti-inflammatory diet, healthy lifestyle and stress management all can prevent or reduce chronic inflammation.

Each cancer is different. Sadly, pancreatic cancer has also struck individuals who were healthy, non-smokers, athletes, and people as young as age 30 to 40. This is a fatal disease. Everybody should keep up greater awareness

In summary

Fighting against pancreatic cancer starts with learning about its risk factors in order to save preventable deaths in the larger population. The impact of pancreatic cancer should warrant public health attention.

Meanwhile, there is hope. And thanks to advanced research and technology that deliver better treatments or promising therapeutic options. So let's also remember *hope*.

The Rule of Three for Pancreatic Cancer Prevention

Pancreatic cancer has a grim reality. To raise higher awareness of this devastating disease among those who are unfamiliar with pancreatic cancer, let me use *the rule of three* to bring pancreatic cancer prevention to light.

Rule #1: Never smoke or drink alcohol, but live a healthy lifestyle.

Cigarette smoking and excessive alcohol intake are well-established risk factors for pancreatic cancer. It's also imperative to sustain a healthy lifestyle, because sedentary behaviors coupled with an unhealthy diet amount substantially to obesity—another major risk for pancreatic cancer. So eat more plant-based foods but less meat or animal fat, stay physically active, and keep a healthy weight.

Rule #2: Prevent inflammation and treat pancreatitis.

Inflammation plays a role in developing pancreatic cancer, and chronic pancreatitis is a known risk factor. In addition, pancreatic cancer is more common among individuals with a history of liver cirrhosis (a chronic liver disease), diabetes, and/or previous surgery to the upper digestive tract.

Rule #3: Keep diabetes at bay.

Type 2 diabetes is closely associated with pancreatic cancer. As the population ages and the obesity epidemic continues, the incidence of diabetes is predicted to rise. People with diabetes are more likely to develop pancreatic cancer than those free of diabetes.

A final point

Still, as is true for other cancers, early detection is always important for combating the pancreatic cancer. This is particularly critical for those with a family history of this disease because the risk can double or triple as a result of familial pancreatic cancer.

In brief, pancreatic cancer is deadly, but you can lower your risk by quitting smoking or alcohol, living a healthy lifestyle, and preventing pancreatitis and diabetes as well. You can also heighten the awareness of pancreatic cancer to save lives.

Why It Is Critical to Prevent Diabetes: Link to Pancreatic Cancer

Preventing diabetes in our own and our families' lives should be of great concern to us for several reasons. One reason is that a diagnosis of diabetes can result in life-altering changes needed to manage the disease. But there is another big reason such a diagnosis is troubling, and that is the urgent need for diabetes prevention because diabetes is a known risk factor of pancreatic cancer.

What is diabetes?

Diabetes is a chronic disease in which the body either cannot make enough insulin (type 1) or cannot effectively use its own insulin (type 2). Insulin is a pancreatic hormone that regulates blood sugar by facilitating glucose (sugar) storage in the cells for energy. When insulin fails to do its job, the levels of sugar in the blood rise.

Type 2 diabetes affects 90 percent of people with diabetes around the world and results largely from being overweight or obese and physical inactivity. High blood sugar levels can lead to long-term damage to the cells and organs as seen in complications like high blood pressure, blindness, kidney disease, and nerve disorders.

Diabetes is a complex condition that requires serious attention and continuous medical care.

What is pancreatic cancer?

Pancreatic cancer is a deadly disease in which cancerous cells develop inside the pancreas, an organ that produces hormones such as insulin and digestive juices.

What is the relationship between the two?

Mounting evidence has uncovered a positive association between diabetes and pancreatic malignancy, although the details of what the exact causal relationship is still remain complex and somewhat inconclusive. Diabetes may be either a symptom or a risk factor of pancreatic cancer. Here are some facts showing the reasons why these two maladies are connected:

- Pancreatic cancer occurs two times more in people who have diabetes than in those without diabetes.
- Approximately 80 percent of patients diagnosed with pancreatic cancer often have a progressive malignancy when a diabetic condition co-exists.
- Patients with new onset type 2 diabetes are at a higher risk of developing pancreatic cancer. When suffering from cancer, they have a worse rate of long-term survival and a higher rate of postsurgical complications.
- 45 percent of pancreatic cancer patients have diabetes, and more than half of diabetes cases are newly developed. Thus, diabetes has been proposed to be a clue for early cancer diagnosis.

Put another way, hyperglycemia, hyperinsulinemia, insulin resistance, and inflammation are commonly seen in both diseases; and have been implicated in the underlying mechanisms that contribute to the development of diabetes-associated pancreatic cancer.

Collectively, diabetes is closely tied to pancreatic cancer and has a negative impact on the prognosis and outcome of this fatal cancer. That is one huge reason why it is so important to prevent diabetes.

Key Strategies for Prevention and Management

Overwhelming evidence indicates that diabetes can be prevented, slowed, delayed, or even reversed through lifestyle modification and/or pharmacological interventions.

To help with diabetes prevention, here are some easy and effective practices you can incorporate into your daily life.

Prevent prediabetes. This can be achieved largely through lifestyle modification with a focus on nutritional diets and physical activity. A healthy lifestyle aids in maintaining a healthy weight.

Keep your blood glucose under appropriate control, especially for people with diabetes. Your sugar levels can undergo fluctuations secondary to daily activities, which creates a difficulty in self-management. But it requires your commitment and skills under the care of your physician or dietician. So adhere to the management strategies with appropriate measures.

Avoid foods high in sugar, calories and fats. Foods high in sugar include rich desserts, candies, ice cream, sweetened beverages, or sugary drinks and fruits packed in syrup. Take this into account. Many processed foods carry excessive sugar and fat. Stick to a low-calorie and plant-based diet.

Drink plenty of water throughout the day. Yes, I mean water, not soda or juice. Staying hydrated is not only healthy but also benefits your body in many ways, especially facilitating the removal of metabolic by-products when hyperglycemia occurs.

Park less, move more. Find ways to be active or functional during the day and reduce the time you spend sitting or resting.

Following these suggestions daily can go a long way toward keeping you free of the plague of diabetes. And oh yes, don't forget to include a network of support (family, friends, and health care team) in your lifestyle adjustment!

Chapter 19

Prostate Cancer

Old Men's and Young Men's Cancer—How to Protect Yourself

Prostate cancer remains most common cancer and the second leading cause of cancer death in men worldwide (next to lung cancer). According to the ACS, an estimated 164,690 men in the United States would be diagnosed with prostate cancer and 29,430 deaths result from this disease in 2018.

Imagine how this may apply to you. About one of six men will be diagnosed with prostate cancer during his lifetime. It's quite somber.

The reality is that men often experience something wrong or annoying physical symptoms but hate to bring them up in conversation. This is understandable, but it can potentially be risky regarding cancer.

First, let me briefly *highlight the difference* between old men's cancer and young men's cancer.

Table 2. The differences between prostate cancer and testicular cancer

	Testicular cancer	Prostate cancer
Age	15–35	50+ (average age of diagnosis is 66)
Location	Outside body, inside the scrotum	Inside body, under the bladder
Risk factors	Race/ethnicity, HIV infection, uncorrected or undescended testicles, injury to the scrotum, family history	Race/ethnicity, 74 percent higher risk in African American men, genetics, family history, hormones, smoking, obesity, inflammation, occupation
Signs or Symptoms	• A painless lump on/in a testicle • An enlarged testicle or swollen scrotum • Discomfort or heaviness in the scrotum • Pain in the abdomen, groin area, or lower back	No sign at an early stage or • change in urinating frequency, urgency, or flow; • blood in the urine; • erectile dysfunction; • pain in the hips or lower back when sitting.
Prognosis	Rare, malignant, but can be treated or cured if detected early.	Common, and can often be treated successfully. Survival rates depend on multiple factors.

How can men be vigilant about their cancer risks? If you are a man, here are twenty things you can do.

1. **Get screened for prostate cancer.** Men older than 50 should consult their doctors for screening, and those having a family history of the disease or African Americans may start as early as age 40. The screenings may include

a digital rectal exam (DRE) and a blood test for prostate specific antigen (PSA).

2. **Detect testicular cancer early.** As recommended, all men should perform their testicle self-examination monthly after puberty and/or have a doctor examine them annually. See a doctor immediately if you find a lump on/ in a testicle.

3. **More active equals more protective.** Physical activity is key to preventing prostate cancer. Some compelling evidence suggests that men who are more physically active have a lower risk of getting prostate cancer. Do whatever works for you—whether that's exercising regularly or becoming physically active in various ways throughout the day.

4. **Maintain a healthy weight.** Obesity is a significant yet modifiable risk factor of cancer. Overweight or obese men are at a greater risk for an aggressive form of prostate cancer.[147, 148] Obesity is strongly linked to diabetes. Diabetes could also influence the association between obesity and prostate cancer, i.e., patients with both obesity and diabetes may have an elevated risk for prostate cancer.

5. **Have more red and green in your diet.** Dietary adjustment is crucial. To reduce the risk of prostate cancer, maintain a diet low in animal fat and high in vegetables, fruits, and legumes. Tomatoes are rich in lycopene, an antioxidant that reduces the risk of prostate cancer. Cooked and processed tomatoes (e.g., tomato sauce) contain high levels of lycopene and are selenium-rich too. Other alternatives are watermelon, carrots, and red peppers. Broccoli is high in cancer-fighting agents (i.e., sulforaphane and isothiocyanates). Regularly eating broccoli can lower your risk of prostate cancer. Other

greens such as cabbage, brussels sprouts, kale, and mustard greens are vegetables rich in indoles, sulfoxide, and 5-methyl-methionine. Together, a "rainbow" plate may have potent anticancer effects.

6. **Consume more fish.** Omega-3 can help reduce your risk of developing prostate cancer. It is found in certain fish, including salmon, sardines, tuna, mackerel, and trout.

7. **Consider biological selenium (not synthetic or supplement).** Selenium, a naturally occurring mineral or essential nutrient as an antioxidant, has anti-inflammatory capacity and may help you fight prostate cancer. Higher selenium levels in the blood are associated with a reduced risk for prostate cancer. However, you'll never go wrong with plant-based foods, particularly those high in selenium, including Brazil nuts, mushrooms, spinach, brown rice, beans, fish (tuna and sardines), shrimp, poultry, and wheat germ.

8. **Reduce meat and fat consumption.** Red meats and processed meats have been linked to a greater risk of several types of cancer including prostate cancer. High dietary fat is also a contributing factor to prostate cancer.

9. **Avoid deep-fried foods.** High-heat cooking (e.g., deep-frying or grilling) generates potential carcinogens such as HCAs and PAHs from red meats, and so does overcooking meat. Studies found that frequent consumption (once a week or more) of certain fried foods (including french fries, fried chicken, fried fish, and doughnuts) is associated with an increased risk of prostate cancer.[149]

10. **Drink more water or tea.** Water helps get rid of toxins, bacteria, and waste in the body. Green and black teas contain potent antioxidants and anticancer agents such as polyphenols.

11. **Drink coffee daily.** Coffee provides a beneficial effect on fighting cancer, according to Harvard researchers. They found that men who drank three to five cups of regular or decaf coffee are 59 percent less likely to develop advanced prostate cancer than those who eschewed the brew. Coffee helps boost metabolism and reduce the risk of cardiovascular diseases.

12. **Be wary about supplements.** There is no clear evidence that any vitamin or herb supplements prevent testicular or prostate cancer. Again, I stress that currently no specific vitamins, minerals or other supplements have been conclusively reported to prevent prostate cancer in humans. Plus the ingredients of supplements are not all regulated.

13. **Listen to your body and talk to your doctor.** If you experience pain in your groin area or lower back, a change in urination (frequency, urgency, flow, or pressure), difficulty urinating or if you see blood in your urine or semen, never ignore these warning signs.

14. **Quit smoking and avoid alcohol.** Smoking is a primary risk factor for lung cancer, but also contributes to several other cancers including prostate cancer. Heavy alcohol consumption increases the risk of prostate cancer at any age.

15. **Limit radiation exposure (except necessary therapy).** Keep your cell phones away from your pants if possible. Cell phones emit RF radiation, a possible human carcinogen.

16. **Enjoy fun for life.** A healthy lifestyle doesn't need to come with boredom. You can exercise, have sex, and watch TV as long as it's not too much. Instead of chips

and popcorn while watching TV, eat a big plate of fresh veggies and fruits.

17. **Prevent inflammation and infections.** Chronic inflammation has been linked to many human cancers. Some viral or bacterial infections are also of carcinogenic potentials.

18. **Avoid or minimize your exposure to environmental pollutants and carcinogens.** Steer clear of carcinogens from all sources, including synthetic household cleaners, artificial sweeteners, processed food products, polluted air, etc.

19. **Ensure you get enough sleep.** Dream sweet dreams. Studies show that sleep deprivation has a powerful influence on a risk for some medical conditions, including infectious disease and cancer. Minimize the exposure to artificial light at night to avoid circadian disruption, as the IARC has concluded that shift work that involves circadian disruption is probably carcinogenic to humans [Group 2A].[150]

20. **Treat an enlarged prostate (benign prostatic hyperplasia or BPH).** There are effective drugs available.

I'd also like to emphasize the following preventive measures for testicular cancer:

• Prevent and treat viral infections. Men with HIV or AIDS have an increased risk of developing testicular cancer. Take a blood test for HIV antibodies, noting that HIV-infected individuals can remain symptomless for years. The good news is that new drugs are available to treat HIV infection effectively.

- Avoid injury to the scrotum.
- Make a healthy diet and lifestyle your priority as early as possible in life. That will lower your cancer risk and help you build up a strong immune system to fight cancer.

Noteworthy is that the two types of men's cancer are highly treatable, but it requires being diligent with screening and early detection.

Finally, ladies, let's encourage the men in our lives to take actions for a healthy lifestyle and cancer protection.

Chapter 20

Skin Cancer

First of all, the skin is an organ—the human body's largest one. It functions as a physical barrier, protects us from injury, infection, variation in temperature, the sun's UV rays, and chemicals. Therefore, it deserves our attention and care.

Skin cancer remains one of most common cancers in the United States, and melanoma is the most malignant and deadest type. According to the WHO, 2 to 3 million nonmelanoma skin cancers and 132,000 melanoma cases occur worldwide each year, and the global prevalence of melanoma continues to increase.

Sun worshippers or beach enthusiasts largely represent a lifestyle or culture, especially among younger populations. At these ages most people don't seriously consider skin cancer a threat as the disease typically doesn't show up until the later stage of life. However, what people don't realize is that the sun-worshipping lifestyle makes young people more vulnerable because they collect what was once a lifetime of sun damage in a relatively short time period.

According to the ACS, "The risk of melanoma increases as people age. The average age of people when diagnosed is 63. But melanoma is not uncommon even among those younger than 30."

Fortunately, skin cancer is one of the most preventable types of cancer. It's easy to avoid the sun because more than 90 percent of skin cancer is caused by excessive or unnecessary exposure to the sun. The sun's UV radiation is a known carcinogen.

Risk factors of skin cancer

1. Lifestyle factors

☐ Overexposure to UV or sunlight
Excessive or long-term exposure to the sun's UV rays increases an individual's chance of developing skin cancer.

☐ Exposure to artificial UV, tanning lamps and tanning beds
Tanning devices give out UV and the experience with it increases skin cancer risk. Tanning beds have been classified as "Group 1 carcinogen to humans" by the IARC.

☐ Tobacco smoking
People who smoke or chew tobacco have a higher risk of developing skin cancer in the mouth or throat.

2. Personal, medical, genetic, and/or ethnicity factors

☐ Fair-skinned white people with freckles
These individuals are sensitive to sunburn, and this increases their skin cancer risk.

☐ Color of the skin
Non-Hispanic/Latino Caucasians have the highest risk of developing skin cancer. They are also at a significantly higher lifetime risk of getting melanoma.

☐ Older age
The older you get, the higher your chance of developing skin cancer.

☐ Previous sunburns or skin lesions
Sunburns, especially blistering sunburns and precancerous skin lesions (such as actinic keratoses), all put one at a higher risk.

☐ Moles
Individuals with a larger number of moles are at an increased risk.

☐ A personal history of skin cancer

☐ A family history of melanoma or skin cancer

☐ Childhood cancer treatment
Childhood cancer survivors have a higher risk of developing skin cancer, especially a greater risk among those treated with radiation.[151] That's why it's important to check their skin on a regular basis, particularly in the areas that received radiation, in addition to applying sun protection measures.

☐ Patients who undergo organ transplant
These people are at a greater risk because of a weakened immune system from immunosuppressants.

3. **Environmental factors**

☐ Outdoor workers with excessive UV exposure on the job

☐ Occupational exposure to arsenal, coal tar or certain chemicals during manufacturing processes

☐ Occupational exposure to high doses of UV radiation or ionizing radiation

☐ Geographic locations
People who frequent or live in sunny climates at high altitudes (where UV rays are more powerful) are exposed to more UV radiation.

Occupational exposure is often overlooked, and its potential consequences are influenced by various environmental factors and individual susceptibility. Overall, outdoor workers and certain occupational employees are vulnerable to developing skin cancer.

Skin cancer greatly affects the quality of life, and it can be disfiguring or even deadly.

How to Identify Warning Signs of Skin Cancer

To minimize your risk of developing skin cancer, the best course of action is to know your skin well and exam it regularly. Early detection is crucial, especially because some common types of skin cancer are curable.

Skin cancer can occur just about anywhere on the skin, but most often on the areas exposed to the sun—the scalp, neck, face, lips, ears, arms, hands, and legs. It can also appear in odd places, such as between your toes, underneath your nails, and even around your genitals. With that in mind, here is what you should look out for, particularly regarding moles, bumps, or spots on the skin.

There is a simple ABCD rule of thumb to start with.

Asymmetry: Is there a different appearance on one half compared with the other?

Border: Do the moles or bumps have an irregular border or ragged edges?

Color: Does the color appear uneven? Has it changed over time? Is it a combination of more than one color?

Diameter: Are there any new spots, or any growing bigger than 5 mm or 0.25 inch (approximately size of a pencil eraser)?

Other characteristics or features include the following:

Fluid: Are there signs of fluid or blood?

Texture: Is the area scaly and hard, or is there any scaly patch of skin that's not soothed by lotion or other remedies?

Height: Is there an uneven surface or bumpy appearance?

Pain: Have the sores failed to heal after a week or two?

Overall, look for evolution or progression. Are there any changes in shape, size, border, color, and/or surface?

What to do next?

If you notice any of the previously outlined signs, check with your doctor or dermatologist to find out whether it's a benign growth or cancer. When necessary, the staff will perform a biopsy. It is always safe to schedule an annual screening for skin cancer.

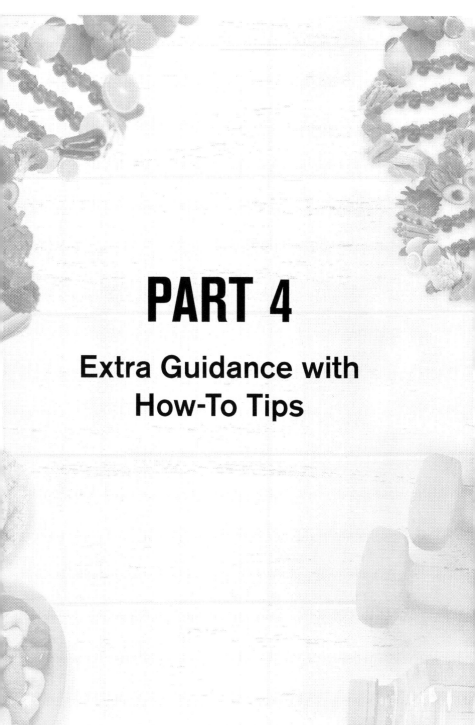

PART 4

Extra Guidance with How-To Tips

How to Integrate Vascular Health and Cancer Prevention

For those who may be unaware of what cancer and heart disease share in common, the outlined contents hitherto have hopefully educated you to some extent. I'd like to elaborate more though. When I started the website CancerPreventionDaily.com and shared my vascular research expertise, I had a well-thought-out approach to maximize heart health benefits along with cancer prevention. To put it simply, there are many practices that will help you tackle two illnesses (cancer and cardiovascular disease).

First, let me ask you this: *Do you know if you have peripheral vascular diseases (PVD) or not?* Millions of people in the United States are suffering from PVD and don't even know it. *What does that have to do with cancer prevention?* Please read on.

What is PVD, and what is PAD?

Almost everyone knows about atherosclerosis. Well, PVD is one of the major clinical complications of atherosclerosis. It affects blood vessels outside the heart and brain (i.e., those of your body's extremities).

When PVD only develops in the arteries, it is usually called peripheral arterial disease (PAD), which results in reduced blood flow to the lower extremities. PAD is predominantly caused by the buildup of fatty plaque in small arteries, leading to the narrowing of these arteries, blockage of blood flow from the heart to the legs, and a higher risk for cardiovascular events. Thus, the hallmark of PAD is extreme pain or painful cramping in the legs. Without appropriate care or treatment, PAD can also worsen the quality of life, cardiovascular morbidity and mortality.

However, many folks with PAD may experience no symptoms. That is why it is important to raise public awareness.

PAD and aging

PAD is neither a men's nor a women's disease—it is more of an aging disease. According to the NIH and CDC, one in every 20 Americans aged 50 and older has PAD, and approximately 12 to 20 percent of people older than age 60 have it. By age 80, 20 to 25 percent of Americans have PAD. It's also a global ailment, because about 20 million people in the United States and more than 200 million individuals worldwide are suffering from PAD.

What are risk factors for PAD?

So far, we have covered two already, namely atherosclerosis and aging. Other risk factors include smoking, diabetes, high blood pressure, high or abnormal cholesterol, hyperhomocysteinemia, being overweight or obese, stress, and a family history of high cholesterol, high blood pressure, or cardiovascular disease (stroke, coronary artery disease, or PVD).

How does PAD awareness relate to cancer prevention?

Table 3. Risk factors that cancer and PAD have in common

Risk Factors	Cancer	PAD
Aging	✓	✓
Tobacco smoking	✓	✓
Obesity	✓	✓
Junk foods / Poor diet	✓	✓
Inflammation	✓	✓ an inflammatory disease
Being physically inactive	✓	✓
Diabetes	✓	✓
High blood pressure, Abnormal cholesterol	+/-	✓
Stress	✓	✓
Hormonal imbalance	✓	-

What are the takeaways?

1. PAD is underdiagnosed and there is a lack of public awareness, but its incident rates increase with age at a disturbing pace.
2. PAD is a chronic inflammatory condition that impairs arterial functions. A valuable and durable approach for prevention is to reinforce the use of diet therapy and weight management.
3. You should make a cancer-prevention lifestyle your priority. Lifestyle modification is one of the keys to preventing PAD as well as cancer.

The message is clear. Take action using the five-second rule, meaning do it now. Whether you consult with your physician or change one unhealthy lifestyle habit, you take one small step at a time.

How to Avoid Too Little or Too Much of Vitamin D

Vitamin D is known for its critical role in forming and maintaining strong, healthy bones. Additionally, it links to a broad spectrum of health benefits, such as those for cardiovascular and neurological functions. Most of us mainly acquire vitamin D from exposure to sunlight. However, the sun's UV rays can cause skin cancer. Does this sound confusing?

Let's talk about some solutions to this problem (i.e., how to make sure you get enough vitamin D for your health but not too much).

How much do we need?

For the general population, the recommended amount of vitamin D daily intake for an individual aged one to seventy is 600 IU. This amount can be increased to 800 IU per day for those older than seventy years. It's important to know that the recommendations are made based on an assumption of minimal or no sun exposure.

How do you get adequate vitamin D?

You get it from the sun but with sun protection.

The most beneficial effect of sun exposure is the production of vitamin D in the skin. However, it is essential to practice sun care and protection. I've published several blogs covering various strategies and tips for sun protection. You can use these resources.

Because UV radiation from the sun can cause skin cancer and because there are other sources where you can acquire vitamin D safely and inexpensively, let's look at how to meet your needs through daily diet and if necessary, vitamin supplements.

You get it from food.

Foods rich in vitamin D include fish (especially swordfish, salmon, and tuna), beef liver, milk fortified with vitamin D, yogurt, cereal, and orange juice fortified with vitamin D. You can integrate these foods into your diet intentionally.

You get it from supplements.

Vitamin D3 (cholecalciferol) is the natural form of vitamin D produced in the skin after sun exposure. It is available as a single ingredient in an over-the-counter vitamin supplement, and it's also commonly incorporated into calcium supplements and multivitamins.

However, take caution with this approach. Excessive vitamin D intake may have unfavorable or even detrimental effects. Following your physician's direction, you can safely use the supplement to correct low vitamin D levels, in order to reduce morbidity and mortality of cardiovascular disease.

Words of wisdom

Vitamin D deficiency can cause health problems, but vitamin D overdose can cause intoxication, including hypercalcemia, renal and hematologic abnormalities. Never take a large dose of vitamin D to prevent cancer since the evidence is inconsistent and inconclusive.

In summary

Sensible sun exposure, certain foods fertile with vitamin D, and required vitamin D supplementation should help improve your vitamin D status, not only bettering bone health but lowering your risk for developing or dying of cancer.

How to Consume Enough Fiber Daily for Cancer Prevention

Imagine fiber's tale. "I am a fiber, and my nickname is Tough Carb. Together with my sibling soluble and insoluble kinds, I am largely wrapped up in foods like fruits, vegetables, and whole grains. Passing through your body, I bind with fats, help nutrients get better absorbed, move the bulk through the intestines, and promote faster traffic to eliminate the waste your body doesn't want. Finally, I still survive, remaining unbroken."

What a fabulous job done by this personal health care agent! Well, I have more good news for you. Research indicates that a diet high in fiber can lower colon cancer risk. Specifically, every 10 grams of daily fiber intake reduces the risk of colon cancer by 10 percent.

But how much fiber do you need each day, and how can you meet your goal to prevent colon cancer? Here I offer five meal strategies that can help you effortlessly incorporate fiber into your daily diet and support the healthier, happier colon.

How much fiber do we need?

It is recommended that we eat 25 to 35 grams of fiber per day. Does that sound difficult? Don't worry. As a rule of thumb, consume at least five servings of fruits and vegetables, and three servings of whole grains each day. This principle is based on the fact that fiber is abundant in whole grains, fruits, vegetables, nuts, and legumes.

How do you integrate 25 to 35 grams of fiber into your diet on a daily basis?

Here are five meal strategies to get your 25 to 35 grams each day with ease.

Breakfast

Eat oatmeal or high-fiber cereal, fiber-rich bread, or English Muffins, and add fruits.

Breakfast is the most important meal of a day. However, many people skip it. Think about this. A cup of rolled oats (dry) contains nearly 10 grams of fiber, and Quaker Instant Oatmeal (3 grams of fiber per pack) is also available in all grocery stores. So if you have two packages of oatmeal (6 grams of fiber), a slice of whole wheat bread (5 to 6 grams of fiber per slice, depending on brands), and add some fruits like berries, bananas, or raisins to your cereal or oatmeal (extra 1 to 2 grams of fiber), you've got a nice jump-start, and it's not hard. Plus fiber can boost your energy for a fantastic day ahead!

Lunch

Eat plenty of veggies and beans. Use whole wheat or whole grain bread to make your sandwiches. Have an apple as a part of salad or dessert. Broccoli, a great anticancer food, holds a good supply of fiber (4 grams per half cup raw, 5 grams in four spears frozen, and 9.3 grams per cup fresh and cooked). Beans and fish (especially salmon) are also excellent protein sources to replace other meats.

Dinner

Eat whole wheat pasta, brown rice, or potato (with the skin) plus a variety of vegetables and olive oil. Add beans to your soup. Did you know cooked black beans contain 19.4 grams of fiber per cup? How about whole wheat pasta with chicken and colorful veggies?

Snacks

Take all-bran, multigrain crackers or high-fiber bars, fresh or dried fruits, as well as nuts and seeds when you are on the go. Figs are one of the highest sources of fiber. Try whole wheat fig bars.

Drinks

Drink more fruit/veggie juice (which is rich in fiber). I'm talking about the homemade ones, not those densely sweetened at the market.

Eventually, it's your choice to include the foods you desire. But the key is to eat a lot of fiber-rich foods (i.e., plant-based food).

Some folks think that healthy foods taste boring, especially those from the grocery stores. I sympathize with that. However, you can get fresh fruits and vegetables from your local farmers' market. Those foods are yummy and refreshing!

As a final note, a balanced, fiber-rich diet is not the only tool to prevent colon cancer. Your exercise should go hand-in-hand with nutrition.

A Cancer-Protective Salad—How to Combine Beneficial Foods

A cancer-protective salad is a colorful one composed of immune-boosting foods and cancer-fighting antioxidants. Here's how you can prepare it.

1. **Use green leafy veggies as a base**. Use spinach, romaine lettuce, kale, or a combination of any leafy greens.

2. **Build on colors**. Use broccoli, tomatoes, onions, mushrooms, or carrots. Fruits such as peach, orange, or grapes are welcome mixers.

3. **Include cancer-fighting proteins**. Use chicken or fish (e.g., salmon). In addition, beans, eggs (hard-boiled and then sliced or diced), nuts and seeds can be good choices for vegetarians.

4. **Mix with antioxidant-rich ingredients**. Use avocado, olive oil, minced garlic, or even lemon. Red wine vinegar or freshly ground pepper can also be used.

5. **Garnish with healthy herbs**. Use basil, chives, rosemary, or any your favorites, whether fresh or dried. They go with the salad components easily. Don't have herbs? Sprinkle a few pieces of green onions.

6. **Add tasty tricks**. Don't forget raisins. They can be an appetizing trick! Alternatively, add grapes for natural sweetness. They are much healthier than synthetic sweeteners and refined sugar.

Can you see this salad adopting or embracing beauty, simplicity and wellness in one dish?

You might say, "Oh, I know this. I eat that and that." Surely, many people know it, but amazingly, many more people load their salads with processed red meat, cheese, unhealthy or fatty dressing, and much worse, salt. Knowledge without action is powerless.

Again, here are the key differences that make this salad cancer-protective and delicious.

- There's a cancer-fighting synergy from various foods.
- The fiber-rich diet reduces your risks of cancer and heart diseases.

- You can make any wise substitutions in ingredients.
- You maintain healthy cooking and preparation habits.

Here's a lunch or dinner recipe. By adding whole wheat pasta to it, the colorful dish turns into your time-saving meal with heart-healthy and cancer-protective benefits!

Together, all the merits are very much in your favor. Beyond doubt—with a few personal tweaks—you can transform this happy combination into a dish of nutritional wonder.

How to Replace SAD with HAD for Colon Health

Did you know an estimated 30 to 50 percent of colorectal cancer cases worldwide may be attributed to diet and nutrition? Do you want to learn how to make your diet effectively fight colorectal cancer?

Let me share with you the top ten ways to eat healthful foods that can reduce your risk of colon cancer.

Today many Americans stuff themselves with the standard American diet (SAD), preferring food rich in red or processed meats, processed or refined food products, high-fat, high-sugar, high-calorie, high-salt, low-fiber foods, and less fruits and vegetables. SAD is tightly linked to many chronic illnesses such as coronary heart disease, diabetes, strokes, and various cancers, including colon cancer.

Here is a solution to this fatal problem. Replace SAD with a healthy anticancer diet (HAD). In contrast to SAD, HAD features a plant-based diet with an abundance of fruits and vegetables, foods rich in fiber, micronutrients and whole grains, but low in sugar, salt, fat and calories, and with little or limited red and processed meats.

Here are the top ten ways to replace SAD with HAD for preventing cancer:

1. **Replace red meat with white meat, fish, and beans.** Red meat contains much more animal fat than poultry and fish do. Convincing evidence shows that a diet high in animal fat is a risk factor for colon cancer and other cancers. As an alternative to meat products, a variety of beans provide not only nutritious dietary proteins but also heart-healthy antioxidants.

2. **Replace processed food products with fresh or frozen fruits and vegetables.** Processed products are more inflammatory yet less nourishing foods often packed with bad fats, excess salt and sugar, refined carbohydrates, and carcinogenic additives or chemicals. These hidden hazards come in fast food or in boxed, bagged, canned, and frozen/refrigerated forms. The only merit they have is convenience. Therefore, avoid or limit processed foods.

3. **Replace high-fat food with smart-fat food.** Your body needs fat to maintain some tissue functions, provide energy, and deliver fat-soluble vitamins. However, you do need to be smart about dietary fat. Healthy fats come from sources such as olive oil, avocado, omega-3 fatty acids (e.g., salmon), and various nuts.

4. **Replace high-calorie with low-calorie intake.** Caloric excess may promote systemic inflammation, which is a risk factor for cancer. Foods with low-calories include beans, green leafy veggies, broccoli, brussels sprouts, tofu, whole wheat varieties (e.g., bread, pasta or spaghetti), and fat-free yogurt.

5. **Replace low-fiber food with high-fiber food.** A waste-loaded or toxic colon may overstrain your immune

system. Dietary fiber is a strong helper in cleaning up your bowels and fighting off colon cancer. So consume various foods high in fibers on a daily basis, including berries (raspberries, blueberries, and strawberries), apples, pears, prunes, nuts, veggies like celery and sweet potatoes, black beans, whole wheat, whole bran, and oatmeal. Most high-fiber foods are also low-calorie and low-fat.

6. **Replace salt with herbs, spices or other natural ingredients.** Balanced natural foods have their flavors. Limiting salt without sacrificing flavor is not as hard as you imagine. For example, my taste is light, and so are most of my family members. Salt is not our friend at the table. With a mix of herbs, green onions, ginger, garlic, and sometimes raisins (natural sweet), our food doesn't taste boring.

7. **Replace fast food with plentiful fruits, vegetables and healthy snacks.** Studies found that eating at fast-food restaurants is associated with higher fat and lower vegetable intakes. To ward off colon cancer, try frozen veggies and fresh ones as a perfect alternative to fast and convenient food!

8. **Replace refined foodstuff with whole grains.** Eat whole wheat bread instead of white or refined items, and have brown rice instead of white rice.

9. **Replace sugar-dense soda and soft drinks with tea or fresh fruit/veggie juice.**

10. **Replace flavored juice with just water.** Research findings reveal a viable association between sufficient water intake and reduced colon cancer risk. Sure enough, water is vital for health and life, period.

Overall, practicing these simple steps can make a huge difference in your colon health and lead to great rewards.

Overall message

Colon cancer is primarily a diet-linked disease. Health-harming food is profitable for the food industry but not productive and beneficial for your life. To prevent colon cancer, change your eating habits now. It's in your power.

How to Control Indoor Dust

Many people are aware of health risks from exposure to outdoor pollution or sources like cigarette smoke, but many remain ignorant of health hazards from indoor dust. The following clear-eyed perspectives may upgrade your alertness.

What can indoor dust do to your body?

On the surface, dust may seem trivial, more of an annoyance than a health risk. However, think about it carefully. Dust contains various harmful substances, such as bacteria, viruses, mold, lead, endocrine disrupters, and cancer-causing chemicals. Because indoor environments have limited volume of air, low levels of dust and pollutants can make up higher concentrations of these particles per breath, contributing to a higher level of hazard to the human body.

The most vulnerable are young children. They spend a lot of time indoors, often at floor level, playing and putting toys or objects in their mouths. They may swallow indoor dust via a hand-to-mouth behavior as they play on the floor, and they may become exposed to harmful chemicals in the dust as a result. This reality coupled with physiological factors, including a smaller body size and an immature immune system, makes children particularly at risk for the dangerous effects of indoor pollutants.

How can you reduce health risks from indoor dust?

Fortunately, we can control indoor dust. Spring-cleaning is an excellent opportunity to do so. However, it shouldn't be the only time. Here are seven simple yet effective ways to control dust and pollutants in your home.

1. *Use a wet cloth instead of dry-dusting.*
2. *Leave your shoes near the door.* Compelling studies have revealed that most floor dust is actually tracked in from the outside and shoe bottoms often contain potentially harmful substances including bacteria.
3. *Regularly replace filters* on heating and air-conditioning systems. The filters help remove dust from indoor air as long as they are cleaned, well maintained and periodically replaced.
4. *Install an air purifier.* Air-purification devices can help reduce the amount of pollutants present in closed indoor spaces.
5. *Decorate with house plants.* Houseplants not only convert carbon dioxide to oxygen but also absorb some pollutants to make the air cleaner. However, not all houseplants can function efficiently in filtering out pollutants or toxins from indoor air. Make sure you pick the right one.
6. *Open windows, and use a fan when cleaning.* The act of cleaning stirs settled dust into the air. When cleaning, point the fan toward the window or use the fan against the window to blow dust outside.
7. *Change the bags in your vacuum cleaners often.* Vacuum cleaners whose bags are too full will not function

properly, only dispersing dust into the air. That's very counterproductive indeed.

Seven Novel Strategies for Spring (or Anytime) Cleaning to Prevent Cancer

Flowers are blooming and birds are singing as spring arrives after a long winter. *Spring-cleaning* is a buzzword. Some people are excited about cleaning for fresh and renewed homes. In contrast, others see spring-cleaning as a daunting task and feel overwhelmed even just running down a long checklist. Either way is understandable.

Here is the point. Spring-cleaning doesn't have to be a one-size-fits-all approach, and you can gain cancer-prevention benefits out of different kinds of spring-cleaning. You will know why after following several novel, refreshing yet actionable ideas and strategies that I outline here.

Manage spring-cleaning with a workable goal.

You may desire that all rooms and corners of your house are spotless, but it's not a must. So setting a priority (e.g., the kitchen or bedroom) can be very workable, especially when time is not on your side. Furthermore, your goal is more achievable when you make spring-cleaning a family function. A bonus is that working together as a family helps foster responsibility for kids. Of course, it's important to do chemical-free cleaning (e.g., e-cloths, baking soda, and vinegar) if you can.

Clean out junk foods to optimize your heart health and prevent cancer.

Go to your refrigerator and your pantry, and you will likely find foods or drinks containing some cancer-causing ingredients such as the following:

- Trans fat: This increases your bad cholesterol and at the same time lowers your good cholesterol. Therefore, it is not only a double whammy on your heart but also a fireball for inflammatory diseases such as cancer.
- Sweeteners: The commonly used aspartame causes various illnesses from birth defects to cancer.
- HFCS or refined sugar: Cancer cells have a sweet tooth!
- Genetically modified organism (GMO) foods: Although genetically modified foods available in the market for human consumption are generally safe, bear in mind that some of them or the chemicals used to grow them might contain toxic substances and fewer nutrients.
- Processed meats: These contain cancer-promoting agents like sodium nitrite or sodium nitrate and potential carcinogens.
- Canned foods (likely containing BPA): Some of them also contain carcinogens.

Clean mental clutter to ease stress and enhance immunity.

Get rid of stress. Get rid of negative thoughts, worries, and self-doubts. Take a yoga class, a bath, or a walk. Treat yourself to a massage, and go out for lunch or dinner with a friend. Whatever works best as a stress reliever for you, just do it.

Clean the fat in your body to gain long-term health.

Obesity is a risk factor for certain cancers, and it also increases the risk for cardiovascular disease and diabetes. So by promoting fat breakdown, you may compensate certain aspects of obesity that cause health problems. Certainly, you cannot gain a healthy weight overnight, but you do have options to modify your diet and lifestyle. Start with cleaning out junk foods and making these efforts.

- Stay away from high-fat and high-sugar foods.
- Start or stick to a balanced diet rich in veggies, fruits, fiber, proteins, and whole grains.
- Trim unwanted calories and make lower-calorie substitutions.
- Burn some fat by exercising and being more physically active.
- Drink more water or tea instead of sugar- or sweetener-rich drinks.

Clean the indoor air to remove pollutants that cause cancer and allergies.

- Check for and remove asbestos, a known carcinogen for lung cancer.
- Test for the level of radon, another known carcinogen. Increase ventilation in your house.
- Install an air freshener, which is a great aid to cleaning indoor pollutants.

How about digital cleaning?

In this digital age, our lives are influenced by digital devices in many ways. Digital hazards can affect your health more than you may realize. You can help detox yourself from them simply by doing the following:

- Clean your inbox. This can get a jump start on a digital detox. Eliminate all junk mail, and if possible, stop those pesky unwanted emails from arriving in the first place. Delete old and useless emails, and organize your inbox in more efficient ways.
- Clean out all electronic wastes, such as old cell phones or other electronic devices, and take them to a safe disposal location designated by your local government. Donate your old computer to a cause if it's still functional.
- Clean viruses, spyware, and malware that may be in your computer. Back up your files, and organize your passwords. Do whatever you need to in order to make your computer run faster and less vulnerable to cyber threats. It will lower your stress level and make your life easier.
- Clear off untrustworthy online feeds or sources. Shut off the fire hose of false tales and misinformation, which are pollutants to your mind and emotion.
- Keep your bedroom free of iPads, iPhones, and other digital devices as much as you can because they are hazards to your snoozing and health.

Of course, you can do more beyond these lists, but you get the idea.

Oral cleaning and care may often be overlooked. Oral health is closely linked to the immune functions too, so clean the mouth to reduce oral cancer risk. Negligence in oral hygiene is a factor for some periodontal diseases that are both inflammatory and infectious in nature. Make a daily habit of brushing and flossing your teeth. Quit smoking. Avoid alcohol. Schedule a dental cleaning and oral cancer screening.

In brief, I hope these strategies provide valuable insights into some small, easy, and quick steps that you can take toward lowering your cancer risk. Spring-cleaning of the areas outlined here can be a great strategy for cancer prevention and other health benefits.

How to Smile

Is smiling easy or not?

Everybody can smile. It's an ability we're born with. There's no need for training. Yet in our modern world, it's amazing how many people walk around with frowns.

Smiling allows us to spread our happiness. Smiling also stimulates our immune system and relieves stress. When one's life is overwhelmed with stress and negativity, it's hard to smile.

Practicing these tips with the SMILE acronym will help you smile easily.

S is for serve. When you serve, give or help others, you feel good inside and out, and you end up smiling.

M is for manage. Manage stress and control negativity, which will make you relax and smile.

I is for inspire. Aren't we all inspired by people who are upbeat, positive, and passionate? Be the one!

L is for love. Love people, and lighten up the world. What comes back to you is mostly based on what you give out.

E is for enjoy. Life is short, so enjoy the moment. Read, play, or work.

SMILE, and you will end up smiling, thus gaining all the benefits—socially, mentally, emotionally, and physically. You will be on the road to good health and happiness.

Wear a smile and have friends; wear a scowl and have wrinkles. What do we live for if not to make the world less difficult for each other?

—George Eliot

Can you smile at ten people tomorrow?

How to Foster and Practice Gratitude

Gratitude implies both the thankfulness for help from others and a conscious, habitual focus on all positive aspects of life. Counting blessings has a proven effect on the well-being of humans.

Holiday seasons are a wonderful time for love and appreciation, but one could be so easily wrapped up with materials and hectic activities that the individual may forget about gratitude, leading to stress, depression, or other negative emotions. A key ingredient for a happy holiday season or for a good day is gratitude.

Power and benefits generated from gratitude

1. Gratitude helps us appreciate the world and connect with the people around us.
2. Gratitude helps us put things or situations into new and different perspectives.
3. Gratitude helps us refocus on what we have instead of what we lack.
4. Gratitude helps us reduce stress, increase healing, and improve well-being.

5. Gratitude makes us happier and healthier.

Remember that it's not happiness that brings us gratitude; it's gratitude that brings us happiness. There is no reason not to find something you are grateful for on a daily basis. Here is how you do it.

Top ten ways to foster and practice gratitude

1. **Do it first thing in the morning.** As a part of my daily routine, I start each morning with reciting what I am grateful for. It can set a positive mood or mindset for the day ahead. So pray and thank God regardless of any form of religion.

2. **Use visual or decorative reminders.** Items such as photos, famous quotes, cards or posts send messages to you and others, sooner or later, the grateful thoughts will penetrate into the souls and turn to the actions.

3. **Apply all your senses and appreciate what you see, hear, smell, taste, feel, and touch.** Only when you've lost an arm (just one of the two) can you realize how precious it is.

4. **Count blessings with your family.** This gives each member the opportunity to express appreciation for three blessings that he or she experienced during the day, week, or month. This is also an effective way to sow gratitude seeds in your kids' minds. I gave my parents credits for their positive influence on us.

5. **Write thank-you notes** (via cards, emails, or text messages) to people who helped or inspired you and those with whom you enjoyed time.

6. **Say, "Thank you," more often and sincerely.** Do not take for granted any simple things that others do to make your life easier.

7. **Keep a gratitude journal.** There are plenty of tips on how to do so, but the key is to take notes regularly and consistently if not daily.

8. **Practice meditation or yoga.** These activities involve concentration on the present moment without judgment and expectation. You can also focus on what you are grateful for (e.g., pleasant sounds, beautiful views, comfortable posture, etc.).

9. **Replace complaints with thanks.** Whenever you encounter a tough situation in life, even unfairness, be thankful for the learning opportunity. Recalling your difficulties in the past, you'll discover how satisfied you are with what you have.

10. **Act on appreciation by doing somebody a favor or supporting a great cause.** For example, have a kind day by offering random kindness. Hey, we all know that actions speak louder than words.

In the end, gratitude is strongly associated with happiness and well-being. Therefore, let's promote wellness through cultivating gratitude with simple practices regularly.

Mahatma Gandhi said, "Happiness is when what you think, what you say, and what you do are in harmony."

How to Boost Physical Activity—Ten Joyful Moves

During the holiday season, we all tend to eat a lot and watch TV a lot, especially for football fans or other sports fans. To avoid sedentary behaviors and weight gain, here are ten practical moves that will help you maintain a healthy lifestyle and cancer prevention.

1. Take a family walk, whether it is a long stroll at a park or a short one just around the block, or add extra walking by parking a little farther from the stores or malls.
2. Stretch frequently, or move during TV time. Walk up and down the stairs as often as you can.
3. Play a game with kids. It's absolutely fun and invigorating!
4. Dance at parties.
5. Practice yoga together as a family activity. It's cool, and everyone can do it. Your body can tell you what's the best or the most natural position. Inhale to breathe in joy, happiness, and peace. Then exhale to breathe out stress, worry, and negativity.
6. Go to a gym or local recreation center to engage in any physical activity.
7. Go ice-skating outdoors or indoors.
8. Bike, if possible.
9. Visit a museum, and walk more.
10. Keep up your daily exercise routine. Yes, it's a challenge during the holidays. My husband sets a great example for us!

Still feel less interested or less motivated? Connect your activity with something greater than yourself. It could be for getting healthier to see the grandkids' graduations, being happier around the family or being more energetic to help others. You get the idea.

How to Follow Feng Shui to Inspire Your Sun Protection

While many people (especially most men) know that sunscreen is crucial to preventing skin cancer and skin aging, they still don't feel the need to wear it as often as they should—even when going outdoors in the summer days.

It's understandable the dreary but obligatory feeling. However, putting on sunscreen is not a kind of unnecessary chore because accumulated sunburns and suntans can elevate the risk of skin cancer many times.

To protect yourself from the sun's harmful UV rays, I'd like to share a solution here.

What is Feng Shui? What does it have to do with health?

For those who are unfamiliar with *feng shui*, let me explain it briefly. If I translate it exactly from the Chinese language, *feng* means wind, and *shui* means water. Originating in ancient China, the principles of feng shui are based on inner peace, serenity, energy, harmony, and joy. Good feng shui promotes good health, and bad feng shui signifies poor health.

How can Feng Shui optimize your protection and pleasure?

Now we focus on how to practice sun protection from a feng shui perspective. If you go out to enjoy nature or the beach, cheers! Chinese favor mountains and water; as a consequence, they view the natural beauty as good luck. In feng shui, the east, where the sun rises, has good energy; and the rising sun represents a new beginning or new opportunity.

Prepare your outdoor journey by getting your sunglasses and hat ready, applying the sunscreen to all the areas of your body that will be exposed to the sun. Massaging the lotion to your skin can also relieve stress. Subsequently, the sunscreen can prevent you from sunburns and enhance your outdoor experience. In this way, feng shui helps you nurture calmness and wellness.

Next, when you are out, minimize your direct or excess sun exposure. While the sun has very strong energy, remember the importance of balance and harmony. Too much strong sun and heat could make you feel tired or exhausted. Staying in the shade helps preserve your energy. Also consider that the sun does cause skin damage and skin cancer—the terrible aftermath should hold you back from overindulgence.

Feng shui is about taking care of yourself, even when it comes to sun protection and skin cancer prevention.

Eight Natural and Powerful Nutrients for Sun/ UV Protection

Have you ever gone grocery shopping, wondering how to take advantage of natural foods for your UV protection? Or you might just be thinking out loud—*Help me. Help me with a shopping list for natural resources of antioxidants that fight UV and sun damage!*

Hey, this is a smart idea or initiative. After all, UV radiation causes DNA damage, which leads to skin aging and skin cancers. Although the skin holds many protective mechanisms against dangerous UV, the combination of accumulated exposure and UV-induced immunosuppression can overwhelm your natural defense. Indeed, there are a myriad of natural resources for your protection.

To combat UV's harmful effects and strengthen your skin defense, here are eight types of superfood rich in nutrients and antioxidants that provide UV protection.

Carotenoids

Carotenoids micronutrients can scavenge free radicals that cause DNA damage to the skin and protect skin from sun damage and UV radiation. In general, colorful veggies and fruits with bright natural pigments are indicators of carotenoids-rich foods. These include carrots, red, yellow or orange peppers, and oranges.

Lycopene

Tomatoes are a lycopene-rich superfood, and lycopene can neutralize the harmful effects of UV rays by scavenging skin-damaging free radicals. Additionally, tomatoes also contain beta-carotene and vitamin C. In every season, it is so easy and refreshing to include tomatoes in virtually any dishes from salad to pizza and side dishes. Grape/cherry tomatoes can be excellent snacks!

Resveratrol

Resveratrol has antioxidant, anti-inflammatory, antiviral, and antiaging properties. It also exerts cardioprotective, neuroprotective, and analgestic actions. Research shows that resveratrol can regulate cellular activities in response to radiation and thus minimize UV radiation-initiated damage. Furthermore, resveratrol can neutralize free radicals generated from UV rays and counteract their harmful effects. Grapes are a superb source of resveratrol. Other foods containing resveratrol include wine, grape juice, cranberries, cranberry juice, and peanuts.

Flavonoids

Dark chocolate is a wonderful source of flavonoids, which is well known for their protective benefits of the heart and blood vessels. Interestingly, evidence also suggests that dark chocolate protects the skin from sun damage. So give yourself a treat or an excuse to consume it regularly but not excessively. In addition, flavonoids-rich natural cocoa butter helps preserve the skin's elasticity and moisture.

Green tea

Green tea is loaded with polyphenol antioxidants, which have protective effects on UV-induced skin inflammation, oxidative stress, and DNA damage. Green tea is also rich in catechins, which are known to have extremely powerful antioxidant properties. A cup of iced green tea in hot summer days serves as not only a beverage to ensure adequate hydration and promote youthful skin, but also a guard to prevent UV-induced DNA damage and reduce a risk of skin cancer. Green tea can be a great substitute for Coke or other sugar-packed soft drinks.

Salmon

We all know that salmon provides an excellent source of omega-3 fatty acids. However, do you know that salmon helps build your skin defense? Strong evidence indicates that omega-3 essential fatty acids may protect against skin damage and premature aging from UV radiation. This is because salmon also contains astaxanthin, a powerful antioxidant that can scavenge free radicals produced from the skin after sun or UV exposure. Additionally, astaxanthin helps alleviate the pain and inflammation associated with sunburn.

Greens

Go greens! And you'll never go wrong. Green leafy veggies are delicious and nutritious, and they help protect your skin from sun and UV radiation. Greens are the fantastic sources of beta-carotene, lutein, zeaxanthin, and vitamins C and E—a full spectrum of carotenoids, micronutrients, and vitamins.

Nuts and Seeds

Nuts and seeds (e.g., walnuts and flaxseeds) are a rich source of omega-3. Omega-3 fatty acids not only defend your skin against the sun's harmful effect, but also equip you with anti-inflammatory capacity. Sunflower seeds are high in vitamin E, which can also protect against UV damage. Plus nuts and seeds help nourish your skin. A bonus—they are portable snacks!

Certainly, dietary intake of antioxidants in terms of UV protection is considerably slower than the topical application achieved by using sunscreens. However, an optimal supply of natural antioxidant micronutrients can enhance skin antioxidant defense against UV radiation damage, support your long-term well-being, and maintain your skin health and glowing appearance.

I hope that today's grocery checklist is valuable for your UV protection and particularly beneficial for people at a great risk of skin cancer and other cancers as well.

Discover Smart Sweet Potatoes

Let's have a conversation on a traditional holiday side dish—sweet potatoes.

First, why do I call it *smart*? It's a cancer-prevention vegetable. Here are the top three benefits of sweet potatoes.

1. They are rich in beta-carotene, a cancer-preventative antioxidant. Sweet potatoes also contain polyphenol

antioxidants. Antioxidants can eliminate cancer-causing free radicals and protect our cells from damage.

2. They are rich in fibers. Fibers stimulate intestinal movements and reduce toxin retention, thus help defend against colorectal cancer.

3. They are good sources of carbohydrates and micronutrients, so they are immune-boosting.

Here are some good tips for healthy cooking and side dishes.

Instead of deep-frying, bake sweet potato fries. Instead of canned yam, roast sweet potato and turnip cubes, and sprinkle them with dill (or parsley). Grill sweet potato slices/chunks mixed with green onions. Instead of having sugar- and fat-rich desserts, bake a sweet potato cake with cranberries and walnuts (or pecans or whatever's desirable), taking advantage of its natural sweetness.

As an alternative to the well-known mashed sweet potatoes, there are a variety of recipes out there, including cinnamon sweet potatoes with vanilla, garlic-thyme sweet potato rounds, apple-cider-glazed sweet potatoes, and grilled sweet potato with wilted kale salad.

Taken together, sweet potato is a delicious and versatile vegetable with rich nutritional values. It provides a remarkable source of antioxidants, dietary fiber, vitamins and minerals, and exhibits antidiabetic, anti-inflammatory and anticancer activities. In addition, sweet potato can synergistically interact with other nutrients that promote health and prevent diseases. Obviously, sweet potato's abundant supply, being inexpensive and easy to prepare are just the icing on the cake.

Eat Broccoli for Protection from Carcinogens and Air Pollutants

I like the following quotation from Robert Louis Stevenson: "Don't judge each day by the harvest you reap, but by the seeds that you plant." The wisdom applies not only to your life but also to human health and earth health.

I love broccoli. It truly deserves a cancer-fighting food spotlight.

A compound in broccoli called sulforaphane has anticarcinogenic properties. A vast body of literature shows that sulforaphane offers chemopreventive and chemotherapeutic potentials in solid tumors and possibly in blood cancer based on its antiproliferative, anti-inflammatory, antioxidant, and anticancer activities.[152, 153] Specifically, sulforaphane can be a highly promising chemoprevention agent against different cancers including colon, stomach, oral, breast, prostate, lung, bladder and skin cancer.

Recently, researchers have discovered that the same compound contained in broccoli also helps our bodies naturally remove some carcinogens or toxins present in heavily polluted air. These environmental pollutants include benzene, a known carcinogen, and acrolein, a lung irritant.[154]

Let's think about it. Is this a better and safer way for humans to reduce their health risks from air pollution? It certainly is, especially without drugs or chemicals. In this way, a natural product helps the body defend against unavoidable environmental pollutants. Again, it proves that food is the best medicine!

As you may know, the benefits of broccoli extend to various health issues such as preventing heart disease, hypertension, diabetes, allergies, osteoarthritis, and some ulcers as well as skin damage by UV radiation (effective when applied topically).

Broccoli can easily be integrated into your daily diet. You can eat in raw (e.g., salads) or in cooked dishes after steaming, boiling, or quick-frying. You can also mix it in veggie juice or smoothies.

The bottom line is that eating more broccoli can go a long way toward enhancing your nutritional status as well as protecting you from environmental pollutants, cancer, and some chronic illnesses.

Green Leafy Vegetables Help Reduce Cancer Risks

Fruits and vegetables contain a wide variety of potential anticancer nutrients and antioxidants. A wealth of knowledge shows that eating plenty of fruits and vegetables has been associated with a reduced risk for several cancers. Here, let's just focus on dark green leafy vegetables.

The dark green leafy vegetable family includes the following members commonly available on the market:

- spinach
- kale
- collard greens
- mustard greens
- swiss chard
- romaine lettuce
- bok choy

Key cancer-protective factor

Dark green leafy vegetables are rich in folate, a group of water-soluble B vitamins. In addition, leafy greens contain antioxidants such as lutein and zeaxanthin.

Key role in cancer prevention

Folate's primary function is to maintain DNA integrity. Free radicals generated by sunlight, cigarette smoke, air pollution, chemical toxins, infection, and endogenous metabolism constantly attack our DNA and cause much of its damage. Without DNA repair, damaged cells can develop into cancer. Folate can persevere DNA stability by regulating DNA biosynthesis, repair, and methylation.[155]

Let me explain a little bit more about DNA methylation. Plainly speaking, it involves the addition of a methyl group to DNA structure. DNA methylation patterns go wrong in cancer, often causing tumor-suppressor genes to switch off, which occurs in common cancers such as colon, lung, prostate, and breast cancer.

Accumulating evidence indicates that inappropriate diet may contribute to one-third of cancer deaths. Folate deficiency has been implicated in the development of several types of cancer, including cancer of the colon, rectum, breast, ovary, cervix, pancreas, brain, and lung.

Key sources for safe intake

To safely and effectively increase folate intake, you should consume dark green leafy vegetables and other naturally folate-rich foods like asparagus, strawberries, and legumes. Supplements are not preferred as recent studies suggest that an excessive intake of synthetic folic acid (either high-dose supplements or fortified foods) may promote cancer.

So eat a lot of green leafy vegetables every day and transform the "green power of prevention" into your body. Leafy greens are loaded with cancer-protective phytochemicals, antioxidants, and nutrients. Also, you enjoy other health benefits beyond cancer prevention.

What's in a Cup of Tea?

Do you drink tea? What is your favorite tea? How often do you drink it? After water, tea is the most popular drink in the world. In addition to its great variety of tastes, drinking tea has been associated with many health values, including the prevention of heart disease and cancer.

What is the key ingredient for tea's benefits?

It is *catechins*. Catechins make up a potent and effective form of polyphenol antioxidants. Green tea is chemically characterized by its abundance in catechins. According to research analysis, a typical cup of brewed green tea contains (by dry weight) 30 to 40 percent catechins, while an equal amount of oolong tea contains roughly 16 percent and black tea 3 to 10 percent catechins.

What is the science behind tea's cancer protective effect?

Cancer protective benefits of tea catechins have been attributed to the following areas:

1. Their antioxidant activities, which positively impact an ability of the human cells to combat oxidative stress.
2. Their immune-enhancing and anti-inflammatory properties, which improve immune functions through the tea's nutrient absorption and immune modulation, in turn controlling immune cells and inflammation markers.
3. Their promotion of weight management, which works through their effects on metabolism and metabolic enzymes. (Notably, tea catechins intensify fat oxidation

and thermogenesis, thereby helping burn body fat naturally.)

4. Their protection against digestive and respiratory infections, as their antimicrobial effect results in the suppression of pathogen growth.

5. Their inhibition of tumor invasion and angiogenesis, the two processes are essential for cancer growth and metastasis.

There is substantial evidence that green tea holds potential chemopreventive effects on human cancer. Having summarized the findings from a total of thirty-one human studies and four reviews, a literature review concludes that tea consumption is associated with reduced risk for cancers of the colon, stomach, esophagus, pancreas, bladder, and lung.[156] New results also show that high consumption of green tea is closely associated with decreased numbers of lymph node metastases among stage 1 and 2 premenopausal breast cancer patients.

Collectively, green tea consumption lowers a risk for cancer. It's also worth noting that green tea has a protective potential against cancer metastasis.

How to Boost Immune System with Yogurt

Go into any restaurant or watch any commercial for a kitchen cleaning product, and enemy number one will be *bacteria*. From a fear of ingesting these microscopic critters, we want them as far from our food as humanly possible. But did you know that all bacteria are not bad? In fact, strains found in yogurt can actually help you by boosting your immune system. On top of that, yogurt's components aside from bacteria can also assist the immune system. Here's a look at both.

Bacteria components

Lactic acid bacteria (LAB) are commonly used in yogurt production. In the finished product, these bacteria must be alive and present in substantial amounts. Does that sound scary? It shouldn't because they strengthen your immune system.

LAB in yogurt are healthy bacteria, and they keep the gastrointestinal tract free of disease-causing germs. In particular, they can increase body metabolism, promote digestive functions, and facilitate bowel movements. LAB can decrease pH in the colon lumen and change the intestinal microecological environment. Increased amounts of LAB in the intestines can suppress the growth of pathogenic bacteria, thereby contributing to a reduction in infection.

Yogurt's bacterial components play a notable role in the immunostimulatory effects of yogurt. Frequent consumption of yogurt can power up the body's immune response, which in turn stimulates white blood cells such as lymphocytes and macrophage, resulting in their destruction of cancerous growth and/or the ingesting of cancer cells.

Nonbacterial components

Yogurt is a nutrient-rich food containing milk, high-quality protein, vitamins (especially folic acid), and trace elements, all of which are necessary for maintaining optimal immune response. Although milk and yogurt have similar vitamin and mineral compositions, calcium is more bioavailable from yogurt than from milk. Calcium can strengthen the immune system too.

The association with cancer prevention

It's a complex subject. In general, yogurt's beneficial bacteria, any compounds produced by the friendly bacteria found in active yogurt cultures, and other nutrients in yogurt may positively influence the immune system, making it harder for cancer cells to survive. Furthermore, as a fermented food, yogurt naturally contains a lot of probiotics, which can strengthen gut health and digestive functions through modulating the gut microbiota.

In brief, yogurt comprises largely the live microorganisms and the nourishing properties of milk. When combining dietary fiber (a prebiotic source) with yogurt (a probiotic food), the mixture can provide a unique benefit for lowering cancer risk.

Now you can enjoy yogurt with added fresh fruits and seed for your breakfast or snack during the day. Just make sure to consume the yogurt high in protein but low in fat, sugar, and calories.

How to Avoid the Risk of Salmonella Infection

Do you eat eggs? They are nutrient-rich, especial when it comes to vitamin D. Now you know eggs can also be a source of food poisoning. In fact, *salmonella* outbreaks have driven nationwide egg recalls from time to time.

Salmonella infection in humans can become chronic, leading to low-grade persistent inflammation. Chronic infections increase a risk for gastrointestinal diseases, including cancer.

So contamination with *salmonella* is no trivial matter. Here are the top three takeaways from these incidents?

Who is most vulnerable to a *salmonella* infection?

Salmonella infections cause nausea, vomiting, diarrhea, and abdominal cramps, as well as fever. Usually symptoms of infection begin twelve to seventy-two hours after consuming contaminated foods/beverages and last four to seven days. However, some cases can be serious and even fatal.

In particular, the following populations are at high risk: young children, elderly or frail individuals, and people with compromised immune systems, such as cancer patients and those undergoing chemotherapy.

What precautions can you take to eliminate the risk?

Again, the food safety system has failed to eliminate the *salmonella* threat. Therefore, you need to take some precautions to protect yourself and your family from potential contamination or food poisoning. Based on recommendations from the CDC and my own practice, I've compiled the following eggs/poultry safety dos and don'ts.

The Don't List

1. Don't eat raw or undercooked eggs.
2. Don't use raw eggs for salad dressing or homemade ice cream.
3. Don't handle food, especially cooked food or ready-to-eat food, before washing your hands.
4. Don't consume unpasteurized milk or any raw dairy products.
5. Don't eat restaurant dishes made with raw or undercooked eggs.
6. Don't prepare or serve food/drinks for others when you're infected by *salmonella*.

The Do List

1. Do wash your hands methodically after handling poultry and any time before preparing foods, especially cooked or ready-to-eat items.

2. Do thoroughly wash the cutting board, the counter surface, knives, utensils, and containers/plates after handling uncooked poultry or foods.

3. Do separate the cutting board or plates for raw food from those for cooked or uncooked ready-to-eat food to avoid cross-contamination—a practice that many folks overlook.

4. Do throw away any cracked or soiled eggs.

5. Do keep eggs or egg-containing foods refrigerated at 45 degrees Fahrenheit or lower.

6. Do cook eggs until they are well done (when both the yolks and whites are firm).

7. Do judge or determine whether meat or poultry is cooked or safe to eat by a food thermometer when in doubt, not by food color or poking depth.

8. Do make sure to cook any egg mixture (casseroles or cakes/pies) until the center of the mixture reaches a safe temperature level.

Is the *salmonella* infection linked to cancer risk?

The relationship between bacterial infection and cancer is rather complicated in the way that bacteria can either cause one type of cancer or protect you from other types of cancer (or both).

Here we're only looking at the link between *salmonella* bacteria and cancer. It's like two sides of a coin.

There is a close association between mixed bacterial and *salmonella* infections with the carcinogenesis of cancer, particularly gallbladder cancer—a cancer with a poor prognosis. Even though one infection won't get you cancer, repeated bacterial infections or chronic infections may lead to cancer development. Therefore, don't overlook infection.

Conversely, the same bacterium, *salmonella,* has been found as a potential strategy to fight melanoma, the deadliest form of skin cancer. Specifically, research showed that injecting *salmonella* (in a safe form) into cancerous mice and cancer cells from human melanoma increased an immune-initiated killing response to tumor cells through elevating immune surveillance.

In short, food hygiene and food safety measures are always worthwhile for your overall health. As the WHO advocated, preventing infection is one strategy to prevent cancer.

How to Reduce Lead Contamination in Water

What are your thoughts on the lead-poisoning water crisis in Flint, Michigan in the United States? Lead-contaminated water also occurred in various cities across the nation. Are you concerned about the quality of your drinking water? Do you know how lead can impact your body in the long-term? Read on. You'll get an instant and clear idea.

Exposure to lead is a serious public health problem because of its association with numerous damages to nearly every system in the human body and its link to various cancers. Here are ten primary concerns and strategies you need to know.

1. **A hidden fact:** Lead contamination is colorless, odorless, tasteless, and likely symptomless. So it often goes undiagnosed or unnoticed.

2. **Routes of lead toxicity:** Lead can get into your body through the water you drink, the food you eat, and the air you breathe. How can lead get into your water? Your municipal water system or your house may have pipes containing lead or joined with lead solder.

3. **The critical numbers:** First, tap water lead should be below the EPA's action level of 15 parts per billion (ppb) or 15 µg/L. Second, in children (especially those younger than five), a lead level of five micrograms per deciliter (5 µg/dl) or higher in the blood should raise a red flag as the reference level of the CDC recommended public health initiatives. If their blood-lead levels exceed 10 µg/dl, the children can be in serious trouble!

4. **The irreversible health consequences:** Lead is a common occupational and environmental toxin with well-known adverse effects on intelligence, school achievement, and behavior. Lead exposure also increases a risk for a variety of chronic illnesses such as hypertension, heart disease, and kidney disease.

5. **The link to cancer:** Lead is one of the heavy metals that are classified by the IARC as a possible human carcinogen.[20] Lead has been linked to cancers of the lungs, stomach, breasts, and renal cells, although further studies are in the works too.

6. **The influence on generations:** Lead possesses genotoxic effects. Lead compounds can cause DNA strand breaks and interfere with DNA synthesis or repair processes. Excessive exposure to lead is associated with an increase in human chromosomal damage, which can be passed on to future generations.

7. **Drinking and cooking water safety:** Never use warm or hot tap water for drinking, cooking, or mixing baby formula. Flush the cold water system for one to two minutes, especially when the faucet has not been used for several hours. (Otherwise, use the water that's flushed out for other purposes.) Filter tap water for drinking and cooking if you can. It also costs less than buying bottled water.

8. **Children and lead beyond water:** Infants and children are susceptible to lead toxicity. So do test your children's blood lead level. In fact, the biggest source of lead poisoning in children today is dust and chips from deteriorating lead paint on interior surfaces or toys. You should also be aware of pica behavior (especially the ingestion of foreign bodies containing lead), which is a well-established risk factor of lead intoxication in children that may cause grave consequences. Lead is such a ubiquitous environmental toxin widely distributed around the world (e.g., the soil in your kids' playground) that even some traditional herbs (e.g., ayurveda) may contain toxic amounts of lead.

9. **Enough calcium intake:** Lead mainly interrupts calcium-dependent processes and calcium signaling in the cells. So make sure you consume enough calcium and antioxidants from fresh veggies or fruits to help combat the negative effects of lead.

10. **Everybody has a responsibility to prevent water polluting.** Learning from the Flint water disaster, we all need to stay vigilant about protecting clean water sources. If you suspect any change in the water, immediately contact your local public health or water system authority.

Bottled water can serve as an alternative, as the FDA sets specific regulations for it. But take a cautious measure because not all bottled water is created equal and bottled water may contain 40 percent or more of tap water.

How to Build a Brand-New Strategy to Cultivate Healthy Habits

Mahatma Gandhi once said, "Your beliefs become your thoughts, your thoughts become your words, your words become your actions, your actions become your habits, your habits become your values, your values become your destiny."

This wisdom from Gandhi can be applied not only to the sake of inspiration for personal development but also to the development of healthy lifestyle habits. So facing many seemingly small battles in healthy living, let's have a strategy mirroring the quotation.

This strategy is to embrace Gandhi's chain of connections from thoughts to words to actions to habits, which in turn lead to immense value of long-term health benefits.

I've heard people say, "Sugar is bad, but I just cannot control the craving." That's valid awareness. So let's use this case for practice to give you an idea of how the process works.

Next time when you feel the craving for sugar or sugar-rich food, try the following steps:

1. **Think**. Consider the fact that sugar doesn't feed nutrients to my body but gives fuel to cancer.
2. **Tell**. Talk out loud. You can say, "I can pass it up," or, "I want to protect my health and starve cancer."
3. **Take actions**. Do something right away to counteract the urge for sweets, such as take a walk or engage in a healthy activity. Alternatively, if you choose to satisfy your craving, eat fresh natural fruits or fiber-rich snacks as a fix. Then give yourself a pat on the back!
4. **Rinse and repeat**. Each time your craving comes back, recall the progress you've made, repeat your valuable words and practice, and visualize this chain of thoughts,

words, actions or behaviors, and habits connecting with your results (i.e., your priceless health).

Meanwhile, never overlook the fact that stress is dancing on the floor! Because stress often has an influence on overeating or making unhealthy choices, it can make people drink more alcohol, eat more junk food, exercise less, and lose sleep—all of which promote overweight or obesity. It is critical to emphasize that stress affects the network connections in our brain through multiple neurological pathways. Thus, shifting your focus can give your brain a break. Relax. Find something to laugh about or appreciate. Apply stress-relief techniques that work best for you (e.g., meditating, socializing, etc.). Certainly, you can create a chain strategy to reduce stress or go after other roots.

Overall, developing healthy habits can keep your body and mentality vigorous. In the long-term, a healthy mind and a healthy brain guide you to function more effectively as you move toward accomplishing whatever you do.

How to Prevent or Reduce Cancer Diagnostic Errors

Have you or your family members ever gotten a wrong diagnosis from your doctor? Have you heard that a doctor treated your friend for a disease or disorder that he or she actually didn't have? "It is likely that most of us will experience at least one diagnostic error in our lifetime, sometimes with devastating consequences," according to national experts on diagnostic safety.

Imagine you were diagnosed with breast cancer and went through cancer treatment and then found out that the diagnosis was wrong and the treatment should never have happened. That could mean enormous damage from one diagnostic error!

Cancer diagnostic errors can be the most harmful and costly type of diagnostic errors in various ways. As many cancers are complex and multifaceted, a timely and accurate diagnosis for cancer is still challenging. That adds weight to preventing cancer altogether and the urgency of detecting cancer early.

That's why I bring your attention to this issue. A diagnosis is something that's done for a patient (you), and the patient (you) needs to be a part of the team in that process.

Basics and facts

What is a diagnostic error?

The Institute of Medicine (IOM) defines a *diagnostic error* as the failure to "establish an accurate and timely explanation of the patient's health problem(s) or communicate that explanation to the patient."

What is the reality?

40,000 to 80,000 deaths each year are due to diagnostic errors, as various reports indicate. However, national diagnostic safety experts Drs. Gordon D. Schiff, MD and Mark L. Graber, MD, pointed out that the frequency of diagnostic error is in the range of 10 percent.

Does it sound like misdiagnosis happens far more frequently than you thought?

When do diagnostic errors occur, and who may be involved?

There's no doubt that human factors contribute to errors in diagnosis. Studies have found that communication problems are the most frequent root cause of serious events threatening patient safety. Today's healthcare systems are transforming toward not only integrated care practice but also enhanced patient engagement. To this end, everyone is involved.

Specifically, let me bring the cancer diagnosis to the forefront. A delayed cancer diagnosis may occur at various stages of the journey to fight cancer. It could be a delay in

- symptom recognition or interpretation,
- decision or action to seek medical attention (e.g., putting off making an appointment because of fear or feeling embarrassed),
- a care system's scheduling (e.g., not being seen by a doctor in a timely fashion),
- clinical tests or subsequent consultations, or
- receiving cancer treatment.

In addition, putting off doing anything might simply be due to a lack of insurance coverage.

Here is the key point. A delayed cancer diagnosis at an early stage may leave the cancer to progress or spread, leading to limited treatment options. Thus, a delay in cancer diagnosis can have devastating consequences, including poor clinical outcomes and a lower chance of survival.

How can you help prevent or reduce diagnostic errors?

Here are fifteen things you can do to enhance your care with your doctor, medical care team, and healthcare system.

1. Prepare for your visit. Know or collect your medical records, medications, and family history.

2. Remember your screenings, and most importantly, follow up. Having a separate calendar can help you keep in mind.

3. Always bring a list of questions or at least your top three questions when visiting your physician. You can also build your own list of questions with an online tool provided by the Agency of Healthcare Research and Quality (AHRQ).

4. Bring your spouse or a family member to your doctor visit to facilitate communication and/or fill in missing information that might help with diagnosis or treatment.

5. Use technology (e.g., a smartphone) to record the conversation or instructions.

6. Feel free to ask the doctor to clarify terminology or procedure. If you don't understand why a particular issue or test is relevant to your situation, ask about it, or let a family member do so.

7. If you have limited English proficiency, make sure you have a family member or a friend acting as a translator.

8. Participate in a patient experience survey to improve patient safety and care.

9. Get involved in assisting the chain of communication (e.g., in scheduling appointments, visits, follow-ups, etc.) and even questioning an insurance company's billing department if you don't understand a charge.

10. Don't self-diagnose, especially based on online information from an unreliable source. Relying on Dr. Google for medical

advice can potentially make the dilemma of diagnostic error worse.

11. Do keep a diary or inventory of your symptoms for better recollections when needed.

12. Seek a second opinion or multiple consultations on cancer diagnosis when in doubt. The second opinion must be from an expert. Be proactive. For example, what if you have a lump in your breast but get a normal mammogram? After all, mammograms pick up only 80 to 90 percent of breast cancer. So for your safety, you should ask for further screening. You can request a breast ultrasound (sonogram) or even a test with a higher sensitivity like an MRI to ensure accuracy if your physician doesn't order such tests.

13. If diagnosed with cancer, follow up vigorously, and treat any referrals to specialists, tests, or care with urgency.

14. Further the discussion about a potentially discrepant diagnosis or different findings.

15. When you have unintentional weight loss, unexplained pain or uncommon signs, take it seriously, and see your doctor.

Misdiagnosis may not be discovered for years if ever in some cases. That's why I cannot emphasize enough how prevention and early detection of cancer offer clear and significant benefits, especially concerning common cancers (the breast, prostate, colon, lung, and skin cancer).

Although I talked more about cancer, these principles can be applied to any other illnesses.

Actively engage in your health care! Improving diagnosis for patient safety and for better health care is a responsibility of each of us. Doing that alone can save many lives.

How to Engage in Personalized Care for Deadly Diseases

Impact of deadly diseases

Did you know that more than 560,000 Americans die from cancer each year? That means more than 1,500 Americans each day.

More than 2,150 Americans die of cardiovascular disease each day. That's one death every 40 seconds.

Nearly 800,000 Americans suffer from a new or recurrent stroke annually. Someone has a stroke every 40 seconds, and someone dies of a stroke every 4 minutes.

Each cancer is different. No two people have exactly the same cancer. That's how personalized cancer treatment works. New scientific advances allow doctors to match the treatments to the biology of an individual patient's tumor.

Imagine if you or your loved one had one of these deadly diseases. What kind of care and outcome would you desire?

The *good* news is that much energy and effort have been shifted to patient-centered care with a focus on individual needs. This is different from evidence-based practice that tends to focus on populations. Therefore, high-quality care and a good outcome must now be defined in terms of what is meaningful and valuable to the individual patient.

The Institute of Medicine has identified six areas for the quality of care—safety, effectiveness, efficiency, patient-centered care, timely care, and equitable care. As a patient, you are the center of care. That means you need to take an active role in disease prevention and get involved in your care.

Because we've previously covered a great deal about prevention, now I'll touch on a patient's role in a high-quality care. These strategies can be extended to many other conditions, including diabetes, obesity, Alzheimer's disease, and even rare diseases.

Ten strategies to help you embrace your role in today's healthcare

Here are ten strategies for getting involved in your health care.

1. **Know your critical numbers and screening results.** These important results include regular checks for blood pressure, blood sugar and cholesterol levels, mammograms, colonoscopies, bone density scans, and even genetic analyses. These findings are valuable for your primary care doctor too.

2. **Tell your story.** Inform the doctor of what's going on with you in addition to simply answering probing questions. Some details of your pain or discomfort may shed light on your condition and offer a correct diagnosis.

3. **Obtain a good primary doctor and a specialist.** Find doctors who have reputable professional expertise and compassion. You want a doctor who takes time to listen to you instead of rushing through clinical routines.

4. **Always have a list of questions in hand when visiting your physician or specialist.** In case you don't know where to start, the AHRQ and WebMD provide some basic questions about different conditions. During your visit, feel free to ask questions or terminologies if you don't understand or delegate a family member to do so. You

may find that the doctor is only asking the question out of routine. Conversely, you may find out that the issues you ignored might actually be very important to your case.

5. **Avoid medical errors, misdiagnoses, and unnecessary tests.** Hospital infections and medical errors kill 500 people each day. Thus, take safety initiatives to avoid becoming a victim. Communicate with your doctor if you have any concerns. Understand why your procedures or medications are necessary and understand what will happen if you need surgery. Always keep with you a list of medications you are taking.

6. **Personalized medicine starts with individuals and reflects the patient's needs, preferences, and values.** Let's face it. Different cancers need different treatments. Likewise, different patients have different needs. Personalized medicine is characterized as the right treatment for the right person at the right time. It may also encompass a biological therapy that targets specific cells or an interactive approach that requires patients and their physicians to develop customized diet plans and exercise regimes or change unhealthful habits. You play a key role in transforming your health.

7. **Be vigilant for new symptoms or concerns (e.g., the occurrence of fever, falling, pain, or swelling).** If you suffer from a serious chronic illness like cancer and have a weak immune system, you are very vulnerable to any infection or inflammation that may worsen your situation. So take care of your immunizations, your food, and your hand hygiene.

8. **Be proactive and active.** This includes choosing a cost-effective health insurance plan and understanding your coverage. It could also mean checking out where the nearest primary stroke center is in town in case of a stroke emergency because time is critical for surviving a stroke! Or you could volunteer to enroll in a clinical trial.

9. **Self-educate, but be mindful of information sources and respect the opinions of your medical team.** Reliable and accurate medical advice can be difficult to determine sometimes on the internet. Medical issues can involve life and death! Respect and trust your physicians because sometimes what you think you want may not be what you really need. For instance, maybe what you want is an unnecessary drug, but what you really need is the right information or modification of your behavior. So don't measure good care by merely meeting your desires.

10. **Get family and friends involved.** Remember that your health care is teamwork. Although you need to take ownership and get in the driver's seat, you are not alone. Your physicians, care professionals, caregivers, the healthcare system, and your loved ones all take the ride with you.

Finally, being empowered with these principles and embracing your active role will facilitate the high-quality, patient-centered care that your medical professionals strive to provide. They will help you achieve a desirable clinical outcome, leading to better health and more happiness for you and your family.

Epilogue

Love and the War on Cancer

Cancer causes much sadness, pain, fear, and anger. It has enormous devastating effects and impacts the quality of life among those with cancer, as well as the lives of their loved ones, too often by shortening life spans.

The idea of an optimistic outlook about cancer came from promising advances in research and technology for cancer treatment and from the focus on prevention instead of cure. Undoubtedly, the fight is far from over, and for those suffering from cancer, there is still a long journey.

Because of the lengthy discussion to empower a cancer-prevention lifestyle, I'd like to emphasize the healing capacity of love, both physically and emotionally. Let's start with nurturing your body.

When in good health, we may tend to take that fact for granted and pay little attention to our physiology. But we shouldn't do that. Instead we should love ourselves, and that means loving our bodies.

Let love penetrate each of your precious little cells. Loving your body begins by nurturing your treasured cells—the fundamental building blocks of your body. With 37.2 trillion cells in the human body, you love each of them by maximizing nutrients' intake and minimizing damage and inflammation. Subsequently, you boost cellular energy and send grateful signals to each cell. And you let love go in or welcome love by exercising your body in an appropriate way for your condition and age. As a result, you take care of your health.

Let love penetrate your immune system too. That's your first line of defense to ward off cancer. The good news is that you can harness the power of your immune system as an effective immunotherapy to cure cancer. Former president Jimmy Carter is one patient who has benefited from such a cancer immunotherapy.

Let love penetrate your whole body by staying emotionally healthy as well as physically fit. Your emotional health is sustained by engaging in physical movement, mental harmony, social connection, and spiritual joy. It helps you work through life's small ups and downs, as well as bigger challenges or trials. By letting love rule your body, you keep peace, develop beliefs and accumulate values that drive positive healthy behaviors.

Let love diffuse into life and the world. Love is communicated in different ways and is easily integrated into a healthy lifestyle. Generally speaking, love can be exhibited in romance and kind acts, in understanding and offering needed support, and in self-care. Love can mean openly talking about cancer as related to one's fears and anxieties too. Find ways to spread love around you. The world needs a lot of love.

In our quest for cancer cure and care, let's embrace something beyond the torture or pain, something beautiful, a deep human need at both a biological and physical level—*love*. Let boundless love nourish our well-being and boost our quality of life.

Acknowledgments

First and foremost, I want to express my genuine appreciation for the tremendous effort of countless fellow scientific researchers and my colleagues who contributed to the knowledge of this book. Despite my bibliography, I must emphasize that the included list is incomplete. Without their dedication and expertise, my insights and values offered in this book would be impossible.

I am profoundly grateful to Drs. Christopher R. Triggle, PhD, Late John A. Bevan, MD, Paul E. DiCorleto, PhD, Gary K. Owens, PhD, and Avril V. Somlyo, PhD (the world's top scientists in the field of vascular research) for their extraordinary mentorships through sharing their expertise, commitment to excellence and outstanding scientific vigor, all these contributed to the guiding principles that I followed to gain this new expertise area effectively. My enormous gratitude goes out to Dr. Christopher Triggle, an exceptional mentor, for his superb supervision and brilliant advice, as well as his kindness, encouragement, invaluable help and support over the years.

I want to give my special thanks to Dr. Harvey McCloud, PhD for his expert editing, proofreading, and generous help with numerous blog posts—a truly blessed support for the cancer prevention endeavor. To all my friends, words cannot describe how much I appreciate and treasure your friendship, cheers and help in many ways; your supports mean so much to me.

I am truly grateful for the remarkable expertise and valuable suggestions provided by the editorial team at iUniverse, especially by editor Justin D.; surely their incredible jobs made this book better to read. A heartfelt thanks to all with whom I have had great pleasure to work during this project, including check-in coordinators, editorial associates, talented designers, publishing services associate, individuals who have worked on the designing and production of this book, and importantly the publisher. Many thanks to the publishing consultant Eve Carson for being with me from the beginning of this journey and for being very instrumental and helpful.

To my wonderful family with a heritage of kindness, gratitude and love, I am deeply grateful for your unconditional love, tender care and steadfast support, which keeps me going in good or bad times. It's hard to articulate my sheer delight whenever we are together and my dearest bond whenever we are apart. Because of you, life challenges haven't stopped me from achieving my passion and aspirations.

Lastly, I reserve my deepest gratitude for Doug Zukauskas, my great husband. I am immensely grateful for his amazing love, care, encouragement, tireless support, and wise counsel; not forgetting his fun and hearty laughter that amuse our day.

References

1   Weinberg RA. How cancer arises. *Sci Am*. 1996;275:62–70.

2   Hanahan D, Weinberg RA. Hallmarks of cancer: the next generation. *Cell*. 2011;144:646-74.

3   Cooke MS, Evans MD, Dizdaroglu M, Lunec J. Oxidative DNA damage: mechanisms, mutation, and disease. *FASEB J*. 2003;17:1195-214.

4   The Centers for Disease Control and Prevention. Current Cigarette Smoking Among Adults in the United States (2017). https://www.cdc.gov/tobacco/data_statistics/fact_sheets/adult_data/cig_smoking/index.htm

5   World Health Organization (WHO), International Agency for Research on Cancer (IARC). *Monographs on the Evaluation of Carcinogenic Risks to Humans*, 2002, Volume 83, Tobacco Smoke and Involuntary Smoking.

6   U.S. Department of Health and Human Services. *How Tobacco Smoke Causes Disease: The Biology and Behavioral Basis for Smoking-Attributable Disease: A Report of the Surgeon General*. Atlanta, GA: U.S. Department of Health and Human Services, Centers for Disease Control and Prevention, National Center for Chronic Disease Prevention and Health Promotion, Office on Smoking and Health, 2010.

7   Bos RP, Henderson PT. Genotoxic risk of passive smoking. *Rev Environ Health*. 1984;4:161-78.

8   Hofhuis W, de Jongste JC, Merkus PJ. Adverse health effects of prenatal and postnatal tobacco smoke exposure on children. *Arch Dis Child*. 2003;88:1086-90.

9   Power C, Jefferis BJ. Fetal environment and subsequent obesity: a study of maternal smoking. *Int J Epidemiol*. 2002;31:413-9.

10 Anderson HR, Cook DG. Passive smoking and sudden infant death syndrome: review of the epidemiological evidence. *Thorax*. 1997;52:1003-9.

11 Hang B, Wang P, Zhao Y, Sarker A, Chenna A, Xia Y, Snijders AM, Mao JH. Adverse Health Effects of Thirdhand Smoke: From Cell to Animal Models. Review. *Int J Mol Sci.* 2017;18:932-9.

12 Matt GE, Quintana PJE, Zakarian JM, Hoh E, Hovell MF, Mahabee-Gittens M, Watanabe K, Datuin K, Vue C, Chatfield DA. When smokers quit: exposure to nicotine and carcinogens persists from thirdhand smoke pollution. *Tob Control.* 2016;26:548-556.

13 IARC Working Group on the Evaluation of Carcinogenic Risks to Humans. Alcohol consumption and ethyl carbamate. *IARC Monogr Eval Carcinog Risks Hum.* 2010;96:3-1383.

14 Roswall N, Weiderpass E. Alcohol as a risk factor for cancer: existing evidence in a global perspective. *J Prev Med Public Health.* 2015;48:1-9.

15 Boffetta P, Hashibe M. Alcohol and cancer. *Lancet Oncol.* 2006;7:149–56.

16 Rehm J, Baliunas D, Borges GL, Graham K, Irving H, Kehoe T, Parry CD, Patra J, Popova S, Poznyak V, Roerecke M, Room R, Samokhvalov AV, Taylor B. The relation between different dimensions of alcohol consumption and burden of disease: an overview. *Addiction.* 2010;105:817-43.

17 Garaycoechea JI, Crossan GP, Langevin F, Mulderrig L, Louzada S, Yang F, Guilbaud G, Park N, Roerink S, Nik-Zainal S, Stratton MR, Patel KJ. Alcohol and endogenous aldehydes damage chromosomes and mutate stem cells. *Nature.* 2018;553:171-7.

18 Testino G. The burden of cancer attributable to alcohol consumption. *Maedica* (Buchar). 2011;6:313-20.

19 Bouvard V, Loomis D, Guyton KZ, Grosse Y, Ghissassi FE, Benbrahim-Tallaa L, Guha N, Mattock H, Straif K; International Agency for Research on Cancer Monograph Working Group. Carcinogenicity of consumption of red and processed meat. *Lancet Oncol.* 2015;16:1599-600.

20 Cogliano VJ, Baan R, Straif K, Grosse Y, Lauby-Secretan B, El Ghissassi F, Bouvard V, Benbrahim-Tallaa L, Guha N, Freeman C, Galichet L, Wild CP. Preventable exposures associated with human cancers. *J Natl Cancer Inst.* 2011;103:1827-39.

21 Hammerling U, Bergman Laurila J, Grafström R, Ilbäck NG. Consumption of Red/Processed Meat and Colorectal Carcinoma: Possible Mechanisms Underlying the Significant Association. *Crit Rev Food Sci Nutr.* 2016;56:614-34.

22 Kim E, Coelho D, Blachier F. Review of the association between meat consumption and risk of colorectal cancer. *Nutr Res.* 2013;33:983-94.

23 The American Heart Association Diet and Lifestyle Recommendations. https://www.heart.org/en/healthy-living/healthy-eating/eat-smart/nutrition-basics/aha-diet-and-lifestyle-recommendations

24 Stoeckli R, Keller U. Nutritional fats and the risk of type 2 diabetes and cancer. *Physiol Behav.* 2004;83:611-5.

25 Ma J, McKeown NM, Hwang SJ, Hoffmann U, Jacques PF, Fox CS. Sugar-Sweetened Beverage Consumption Is Associated With Change of Visceral Adipose Tissue Over 6 Years of Follow-Up. *Circulation.* 2016;133:370-7.

26 Johnson RK, Frary C. Choose beverages and foods to moderate your intake of sugars: the 2000 dietary guidelines for Americans—what's all the fuss about? *J Nutr.* 2001;131:2766S-71S.

27 Baldo MP, Rodrigues SL, Mill JG. High salt intake as a multifaceted cardiovascular disease: new support from cellular and molecular evidence. *Heart Fail Rev.* 2015;20:461-74.

28 He J, Gu D, Chen J, Wu X, Kelly TN, Huang JF, Chen JC, Chen CS, Bazzano LA, Reynolds K, Whelton PK, Klag MJ. Premature deaths attributable to blood pressure in China: a prospective cohort study. *Lancet.* 2009;374:1765-72.

29 Rochester JR. Bisphenol A and human health: a review of the literature. *Reprod Toxicol.* 2013;42:132-55

30 Seachrist DD, Bonk KW, Ho SM, Prins GS, Soto AM, Keri RA. A Review of the Carcinogenic Potential of Bisphenol A. *Reprod Toxicol.* 2016;59:167–182.

31 IARC Working Group. Some naturally occurring and synthetic food components, furocoumarins and ultraviolet radiation. *IARC Monogr Eval Carcinog Risk Chem Hum.* 1986;40:1-415.

32 Bauer AK, Dwyer-Nield LD, Hankin JA, Murphy RC, Malkinson AM. The lung tumor promoter, butylated hydroxytoluene (BHT), causes chronic inflammation in promotion-sensitive BALB/cByJ mice but not in promotion-resistant CXB4 mice. *Toxicology.* 2001;169:1-15.

33 World Cancer Research Fund, American Institute for Cancer Research. Food, Nutrition, Physical Activity, and the Prevention of Cancer: a Global Perspective. Washington, DC: AICR, 2007

34 Lynch BM. Sedentary Behavior and Cancer. *Cancer Epidemiol Biomarkers Prev.* 2010;19:2691-2709.

35 Ruiz-Casado A, Martín-Ruiz A, Pérez LM, Provencio M, Fiuza-Luces C, Lucia A. Exercise and the Hallmarks of Cancer. *Trends Cancer.* 2017;3:423-41.

36 The American Cancer Society. ACS Guidelines for Nutrition and Physical Activity. https://www.cancer.org/healthy/eat-healthy-get-active/acs-guidelines-nutrition-physical-activity-cancer-prevention/guidelines.html

37 Wolin KY, Lee IM, Colditz GA, Glynn RJ, Fuchs C, Giovannucci E. Leisure-time physical activity patterns and risk of colon cancer in women. *Int J Cancer*. 2007;121:2776-81.

38 Lemanne D, Cassileth B, Gubili J. The role of physical activity in cancer prevention, treatment, recovery, and survivorship. *Oncology (Williston Park)*. 2013;27:580-5.

39 Li Q, Kobayashi M, Inagaki H, Hirata Y, Li YJ, Hirata K, Shimizu T, Suzuki H, Katsumata M, Wakayama Y, Kawada T, Ohira T, Matsui N, Kagawa T. A day trip to a forest park increases human natural killer activity and the expression of anti-cancer proteins in male subjects. *J Biol Regul Homeost Agents*. 2010;24:157-65.

40 Simpson RJ, Kunz H, Agha N, Graff R. Exercise and the Regulation of Immune Functions. *Prog Mol Biol Transl Sci*. 2015;135:355-80.

41 Becker S, Dossus L, Kaaks R. Obesity related hyperinsulinaemia and hyperglycaemia and cancer development. *Arch Physiol Biochem*. 2009;115:86-96.

42 Bandini M, Gandaglia G, Briganti A. Obesity and prostate cancer. *Curr Opin Urol*. 2017;27:415-421.

43 De Pergola G, Silvestris F. Obesity as a major risk factor for cancer. *J Obes*. 2013; 2013:291546.

44 Yiannikouris F, Karounos M, Charnigo R, English VL, Rateri DL, Daugherty A, Cassis LA. Adipocyte-specific deficiency of angiotensinogen decreases plasma angiotensinogen concentration and systolic blood pressure in mice. *Am J Physiol Regul Integr Comp Physiol*. 2012;302:R244-51.

45 Hui Xie, John A. Bevan. Ox-LDL enhances myogenic tone in the rabbit posterior cerebral artery through the release of endothelin-1. *Stroke*. 1999;30:2423-30.

46 Eichhorn B, Muller G, Leuner A, Sawamura T, Ravens U, Morawietz H. Impaired vascular function in small resistance arteries of LOX-1 overexpressing mice on high-fat diet. *Cardiovasc Res*. 2009;82:493–502.

47 Donohoe CL, Doyle SL, Reynolds JV. Visceral adiposity, insulin resistance and cancer risk. *Diabetol Metab Syndr*. 2011;3:12-23.

48 Britton KA, Massaro JM, Murabito JM, Kreger BE, Hoffmann U, Fox CS. Body fat distribution, incident cardiovascular disease, cancer, and all-cause mortality. *J Am Coll Cardiol.* 2013;62:921-5.

49 Pierce GL, Beske SD, Lawson BR, Southall KL, Benay FJ, Donato AJ, Seals DR. Weight loss alone improves conduit and resistance artery endothelial function in young and older overweight/obese adults. *Hypertension.* 2008;52:72-9.

50 Debette S, Beiser A, Hoffmann U, Decarli C, O'Donnell CJ, Massaro JM, Au R, Himali JJ, Wolf PA, Fox CS, Seshadri S. Visceral fat is associated with lower brain volume in healthy middle-aged adults. *Ann Neurol.* 2010;68:136-44.

51 Jagust W, Harvey D, Mungas D, Haan M. Central obesity and the aging brain. *Arch Neurol.* 2005;62:1545-8.

52 Turnbaugh PJ, Ley RE, Mahowald MA, Magrini V, Mardis ER, Gordon JI. An obesity-associated gut microbiome with increased capacity for energy harvest. *Nature.* 2006;444:1027–31.

53 Turnbaugh PJ, Hamady M, Yatsunenko T, Cantarel BL, Duncan A, Ley RE. A core gut microbiome in obese and lean twins. *Nature.* 2009;457:480–4.

54 Buford TW. (Dis)Trust your gut: the gut microbiome in age-related inflammation, health, and disease. (Review) *Microbiome.* 2017;5:80

55 Nagpal R, Mainali R, Ahmadi S, Wang S, Singh R, Kavanagh K, Kitzman DW, Kushugulova A, Marotta F, Yadav H. Gut microbiome and aging: Physiological and mechanistic insights. *Nutr Healthy Aging.* 2018;4:267-85.

56 Oliveros E, Somers VK, Sochor O, Goel K, Lopez-Jimenez F. The concept of normal weight obesity. *Prog Cardiovasc Dis.* 2014;56:426-33.

57 Mann JN, Thakore JH. Melancholic depression and abdominal fat distribution: a mini-review. *Stress.* 1999;3:1-15.

58 Ruchirawat M, Navasumrit P, Settachan D, Autrup H. Environmental impacts on children's health in Southeast Asia: genotoxic compounds in urban air. *Ann N Y Acad Sci.* 2006;1076:678-90.

59 Fucic A, Gamulin M, Ferencic Z, Katic J, Krayer von Krauss M, Bartonova A, Merlo DF. Environmental exposure to xenoestrogens and oestrogen related cancers: reproductive system, breast, lung, kidney, pancreas, and brain. *Environ Health.* 2012;11(Suppl. 1):S8-16.

60 Costello A, Abbas M, Allen A, Ball S, Bell S, Bellamy R, Friel S, Groce N, Johnson A, Kett M, Lee M, Levy C, Maslin M, McCoy D, McGuire B, Montgomery H, Napier D, Pagel C, Patel J, de Oliveira JA, Redclift

N, Rees H, Rogger D, Scott J, Stephenson J, Twigg J, Wolff J, Patterson C. Managing the health effects of climate change: Lancet and University College London Institute for Global Health Commission. *Lancet.* 2009;373:1693-733.

61 IARC Working Group on the Evaluation of Carcinogenic Risks to Humans. Outdoor Air Pollution. *IARC Monogr Eval Carcinog Risks Hum.* 2016;109:9-444.

62 El Ghissassi F, Baan R, Straif K, Grosse Y, Secretan B, Bouvard V, Benbrahim-Tallaa L, Guha N, Freeman C, Galichet L, Cogliano V; WHO International Agency for Research on Cancer Monograph Working Group. A review of human carcinogens—part D: radiation. *Lancet Oncol.* 2009;10:751-2.

63 Murphy GM. Ultraviolet radiation and immunosuppression. *Br J Dermatol.* 2009;161(Suppl. 3):90-5.

64 Sample A, He YY. Mechanisms and prevention of UV-induced melanoma. *Photodermatol Photoimmunol Photomed.* 2018;34:13-24.

65 The Environment Protection Agency. Health Effects of UV Radiation. https://www.epa.gov/sunsafety/health-effects-uv-radiation

66 Hardell L, Carlberg M, Söderqvist F, Mild KH, Morgan LL. Long-term use of cellular phones and brain tumours: increased risk associated with use for > or =10 years. *Occup Environ Med.* 2007;64:626-32.

67 IARC Working Group on the Evaluation of Carcinogenic Risks to Humans. Non-ionizing radiation, Part 2: Radiofrequency electromagnetic fields. *IARC Monogr Eval Carcinog Risks Hum.* 2013;102(PT 2):1–460.

68 Mead MN. Cancer: Strong Signal for Cell Phone Effects. *Environ Health Perspect.* 2008;116:A422.

69 Samaras V, Rafailidis PI, Mourtzoukou EG, Peppas G, Falagas ME. Chronic bacterial and parasitic infections and cancer: a review. *J Infect Dev Ctries.* 2010;4:267-81.

70 Di Domenico EG, Cavallo I, Pontone M, Toma L, Ensoli F. Biofilm Producing *Salmonella* Typhi: Chronic Colonization and Development of Gallbladder Cancer. *Int J Mol Sci.* 2017;18:1887-900.

71 Botelho MC, Alves H, Richter J. Halting *Schistosoma haematobium* - associated bladder cancer. *Int J Cancer Manag.* 2017;10: e9430.

72 Ishida K, Hsieh MH. Understanding Urogenital Schistosomiasis-Related Bladder Cancer: An Update. *Front Med (Lausanne).* 2018;5:223.

73 Dejea C, Wick E, Sears CL. Bacterial oncogenesis in the colon. *Future Microbiol.* 2013;8:445-60.

74 Mármol I, Sánchez-de-Diego C, Pradilla Dieste A, Cerrada E, Rodriguez Yoldi MJ. Colorectal Carcinoma: A General Overview and Future Perspectives in Colorectal Cancer. *Int J Mol Sci.* 2017;18:197-235.

75 Tomkovich S, Jobin C. Microbial networking in cancer: when two toxins collide. *Br J Cancer.* 2018;118:1407-9.

76 Morales-Sánchez A, Fuentes-Pananá EM. Human viruses and cancer. *Viruses.* 2014;6:4047-79.

77 Coussens LM, Werb Z. Inflammation and cancer. *Nature.* 2002;420:860–7.

78 Libby P. Inflammation and cardiovascular disease mechanisms. *Am J Clin Nutr.* 2006;83:456S–460S.

79 Esposito K, Nappo F, Marfella R, Giugliano G, Giugliano F, Ciotola M, Quagliaro L, Ceriello A, Giugliano D. Inflammatory cytokine concentrations are acutely increased by hyperglycemia in humans: role of oxidative stress. *Circulation.* 2002;106:2067–72.

80 Berg AH, Scherer PE. Adipose tissue, inflammation, and cardiovascular disease. *Circ Res.* 2005;96:939–49.

81 White MC, Holman DM, Boehm JE, Peipins LA, Grossman M, Henley SJ. Age and cancer risk: a potentially modifiable relationship. *Am J Prev Med.* 2014;46:S7-15.

82 Zhang X, Meng X, Chen Y, Leng SX, Zhang H. The Biology of Aging and Cancer: Frailty, Inflammation, and Immunity. *Cancer J.* 2017;23:201-5.

83 Aunan JR, Cho WC, Søreide K. The Biology of Aging and Cancer: A Brief Overview of Shared and Divergent Molecular Hallmarks. *Aging Dis.* 2017;8:628-42.

84 Armanios M. Telomeres and age-related disease: how telomere biology informs clinical paradigms. *J Clin Invest.* 2013;123:996-1002.

85 Fulop T, Witkowski JM, Olivieri F, Larbi A. The integration of inflammaging in age-related diseases. *Semin Immunol.* 2018;40:17-35.

86 Kaeberlein M. Longevity and aging. *F1000Prime Rep.* 2013;5:5-12.

87 Irwin MR. Why sleep is important for health: a psychoneuroimmunology perspective. *Annu Rev Psychol.* 2015;66:143-72.

88 Ali T, Choe J, Awab A, Wagener TL, Orr WC. Sleep, immunity and inflammation in gastrointestinal disorders. World J Gastroenterol. 2013;19:9231-9.

89 Noguti J, Andersen ML, Cirelli C, Ribeiro DA. Oxidative stress, cancer, and sleep deprivation: is there a logical link in this association? *Sleep Breath.* 2013;17:905-10.

90 Owens RL, Gold KA, Gozal D, Peppard PE, Jun JC, Lippman SM, Malhotra A; UCSD Sleep and Cancer Symposium Group. Sleep and Breathing … and Cancer? *Cancer Prev Res (Phila)*. 2016;9:821-7.

91 Gozal D, Farré R, Nieto FJ. Putative Links Between Sleep Apnea and Cancer: From Hypotheses to Evolving Evidence. *Chest*. 2015;148:1140-7.

92 Xiao Q, Keadle SK, Hollenbeck AR, Matthews CE. Sleep duration and total and cause-specific mortality in a large US cohort: interrelationships with physical activity, sedentary behavior, and body mass index. *Am J Epidemiol*. 2014;180:997-1006.

93 Godbout JP, Glaser R. Stress-induced immune dysregulation: implications for wound healing, infectious disease and cancer. *J Neuroimmune Pharmacol*. 2006;1:421-7.

94 Yang EV, Glaser R. Stress-induced immunomodulation and the implications for health. *Int Immunopharmacol*. 2002;2:315-24.

95 Flint MS, Baum A, Chambers WH, Jenkins FJ. Induction of DNA damage, alteration of DNA repair and transcriptional activation by stress hormones. *Psychoneuroendocrinology*. 2007;32:470-9.

96 Srivastava KK, Kumar R. Stress, oxidative injury and disease. *Indian J Clin Biochem*. 2015;30:3-10.

97 Adam TC, Epel ES. Stress, eating and the reward system. *Physiol Behav*. 2007;91:449-58.

98 Moussas GI, Papadopoulou AG. Substance abuse and cancer. *Psychiatriki*. 2017;28:234-41.

99 Li JH, Lin LF. Genetic toxicology of abused drugs: a brief review. *Mutagenesis*. 1998;13:557-65.

100 Kamangar F, Shakeri R, Malekzadeh R, Islami F. Opium use: an emerging risk factor for cancer? *Lancet Oncol*. 2014;15:e69-77.

101 Afshari M, Janbabaei G, Bahrami MA, Moosazadeh M. A systematic review and meta-analysis of the odds ratios for opium use and the risk of bladder cancer. *PLoS One*. 2017;12:e0178527.

102 Chan YX, Yeap BB. Dihydrotestosterone and cancer risk. *Curr Opin Endocrinol Diabetes Obes*. 2018;25:209-217.

103 Goldberg L. Possible Health Effects of Anabolic Steroids. https://www.hormone.org/hormones-and-health/steroid-and-hormone-abuse/health-effects.

104 de-Tomás J, Monturiol JM. Is there any relationship between drug addiction and the development of a signet ring cell carcinoma of the stomach? *Rev Esp Enferm Dig*. 2016;108:167-8.

105 Huang YH, Zhang ZF, Tashkin DP, Feng B, Straif K, Hashibe M. An epidemiologic review of marijuana and cancer: an update. *Cancer Epidemiol Biomarkers Prev.* 2015;24:15-31.

106 Underner M, Urban T, Perriot J, de Chazeron I, Meurice JC. [Cannabis smoking and lung cancer]. *Rev Mal Respir.* 2014;31:488-98.

107 Gates P, Jaffe A, Copeland J. Cannabis smoking and respiratory health: consideration of the literature. *Respirology.* 2014;19:655-62.

108 Hashibe M, Straif K, Tashkin DP, Morgenstern H, Greenland S, Zhang ZF. Epidemiologic review of marijuana use and cancer risk. *Alcohol.* 2005;35:265-75.

109 Hashibe M, Ford DE, Zhang ZF. Marijuana smoking and head and neck cancer. *J Clin Pharmacol.* 2002;42:103S-107S.

110 Zhang ZF, Morgenstern H, Spitz MR, Tashkin DP, Yu GP, Marshall JR, Hsu TC, Schantz SP. Marijuana use and increased risk of squamous cell carcinoma of the head and neck. *Cancer Epidemiol Biomarkers Prev.* 1999;8:1071-8.

111 Mehra R, Moore BA, Crothers K, Tetrault J, Fiellin DA. The association between marijuana smoking and lung cancer: a systematic review. *Arch Intern Med.* 2006;166:1359-67.

112 Tashkin DP, Baldwin GC, Sarafian T, Dubinett S, Roth MD. Respiratory and immunologic consequences of marijuana smoking. *J Clin Pharmacol.* 2002;42(S1):71S-81S.

113 Skeldon SC, Goldenberg SL. Urological complications of illicit drug use. *Nat Rev Urol.* 2014;11:169-77.

114 Nelson RA, Levine AM, Marks G, Bernstein L. Alcohol, tobacco and recreational drug use and the risk of non-Hodgkin's lymphoma. *Br J Cancer.* 1997;76:1532-7.

115 Chao C, Jacobson LP, Tashkin D, Martínez-Maza O, Roth MD, Margolick JB, Chmiel JS, Holloway MN, Zhang ZF, Detels R. Recreational amphetamine use and risk of HIV-related non-Hodgkin lymphoma. *Cancer Causes Control.* 2009;20:509-16.

116 Minkoff H, Zhong Y, Strickler HD, Watts DH, Palefsky JM, Levine AM, D'Souza G, Howard AA, Plankey M, Massad LS, Burk R. The relationship between cocaine use and human papillomavirus infections in HIV-seropositive and HIV-seronegative women. *Infect Dis Obstet Gynecol.* 2008;2008:587082.

117 Ropek N, Al-Serori H, Mišík M, Nersesyan A, Sitte HH, Collins AR, Shaposhnikov S, Knasmüller S, Kundi M, Ferk F. Methamphetamine

("crystal meth") causes induction of DNA damage and chromosomal aberrations in human derived cells. *Food Chem Toxicol.* 2019;128:1-7.

118 Lopes CF, de Angelis BB, Prudente HM, de Souza BV, Cardoso SV, de Azambuja Ribeiro RI. Concomitant consumption of marijuana, alcohol and tobacco in oral squamous cell carcinoma development and progression: recent advances and challenges. *Arch Oral Biol.* 2012;57:1026-33.

119 Althobaiti YS, Sari Y. Alcohol Interactions with Psychostimulants: An Overview of Animal and Human Studies. *J Addict Res Ther.* 2016;7:281.

120 Hulka BS. Epidemiology of susceptibility to breast cancer. *Prog Clin Biol Res.* 1996;395:159-74.

121 Flaherty RL, Owen M, Fagan-Murphy A, Intabli H, Healy D, Patel A, Allen MC, Patel BA, Flint MS. Glucocorticoids induce production of reactive oxygen species/reactive nitrogen species and DNA damage through an iNOS mediated pathway in breast cancer. *Breast Cancer Res.* 2017;19:35-47.

122 Russo J, Russo IH. The role of estrogen in the initiation of breast cancer. *J Steroid Biochem Mol Biol.* 2006;102:89-96.

123 Daly B, Olopade OI. Race, ethnicity, and the diagnosis of breast cancer. *JAMA.* 2015;313:141-2.

124 Guillén-Ponce C, Serrano R, Sánchez-Heras AB, Teulé A, Chirivella I, Martín T, Martínez E, Morales R, Robles L. Clinical guideline seom: hereditary colorectal cancer. *Clin Transl Oncol.* 2015;17:962-71.

125 Slattery ML, Curtin K, Schaffer D, Anderson K, Samowitz W. Associations between family history of colorectal cancer and genetic alterations in tumors. *Int J Cancer.* 2002;97:823-7.

126 Thangaraju M, Cresci GA, Liu K, Ananth S, Gnanaprakasam JP, Browning DD, Mellinger JD, Smith SB, Digby GJ, Lambert NA, Prasad PD, Ganapathy V. GPR109A is a G-protein-coupled receptor for the bacterial fermentation product butyrate and functions as a tumor suppressor in colon. *Cancer Res.* 2009;69:2826-32.

127 Singh N, Gurav A, Sivaprakasam S, Brady E, Padia R, Shi H, Thangaraju M, Prasad PD, Manicassamy S, Munn DH, Lee JR, Offermanns S, Ganapathy V. Activation of Gpr109a, receptor for niacin and the commensal metabolite butyrate, suppresses colonic inflammation and carcinogenesis. *Immunity.* 2014;40:128-39.

128 Hardell L. World Health Organization, radiofrequency radiation and health - a hard nut to crack (Review). *Int J Oncol.* 2017; 51:405-413.

129 Gandhi OP, Morgan LL, de Salles AA, Han Y-Y, Herberman RB, Davis DL. Exposure limits: The underestimation of absorbed cell phone radiation, especially in children. *Electromagn Biol Med.* 2012; 31:34–51.

130 Belson M, Kingsley B, Holmes A. Risk factors for acute leukemia in children: a review. *Environ Health Perspect.* 2007;115:138-45.

131 Snyder R. Leukemia and benzene. *Int J Environ Res Public Health.* 2012;9:2875-93.

132 The Centers for Disease Control and Prevention. Facts About Benzene. https://emergency.cdc.gov/agent/benzene/basics/facts.asp

133 Gibbons DL, Byers LA, Kurie JM. Smoking, p53 mutation, and lung cancer. *Mol Cancer Res.* 2014;12:3-13.

134 Abegglen LM, Caulin AF, Chan A, Lee K, Robinson R, Campbell MS, Kiso WK, Schmitt DL, Waddell PJ, Bhaskara S, Jensen ST, Maley CC, Schiffman JD. Potential Mechanisms for Cancer Resistance in Elephants and Comparative Cellular Response to DNA Damage in Humans. *JAMA.* 2015;314:1850-60.

135 Goldman R, Shields PG. Food mutagens. *J Nutr.* 2003;133(Suppl 3):965S-973S.

136 Lam TK, Cross AJ, Consonni D, Randi G, Bagnardi V, Bertazzi PA, Caporaso NE, Sinha R, Subar AF, Landi MT. Intakes of red meat, processed meat, and meat mutagens increase lung cancer risk. *Cancer Res.* 2009;69:932-9.

137 Yang WS, Wong MY, Vogtmann E, Tang RQ, Xie L, Yang YS, Wu QJ, Zhang W, Xiang YB. Meat consumption and risk of lung cancer: evidence from observational studies. *Ann Oncol.* 2012;23:3163-70.

138 Vogeltanz-Holm N, Schwartz GG. Radon and lung cancer: What does the public really know? *J Environ Radioact.* 2018;192:26-31.

139 Rahib L, Smith BD, Aizenberg R, Rosenzweig AB, Fleshman JM, Matrisian LM. Projecting cancer incidence and deaths to 2030: the unexpected burden of thyroid, liver, and pancreas cancers in the United States. *Cancer Res.* 2014;74:2913-21.

140 Amundadottir LT. Pancreatic Cancer Genetics. *Int J Biol Sci.* 2016;12:314-25.

141 Barone E, Corrado A, Gemignani F, Landi S. Environmental risk factors for pancreatic cancer: an update. *Arch Toxicol.* 2016;90:2617-42.

142 Sheflin AM, Whitney AK, Weir TL. Cancer-promoting effects of microbial dysbiosis. *Curr Oncol Rep.* 2014;16:406.

143 Ertz-Archambault N, Keim P, Von Hoff D. Microbiome and pancreatic cancer: A comprehensive topic review of literature. *World J Gastroenterol.* 2017;23:1899-908.

144 Michaud DS. Role of bacterial infections in pancreatic cancer. *Carcinogenesis.* 2013;34:2193-7.

145 Öğrendik M. Periodontal Pathogens in the Etiology of Pancreatic Cancer. *Gastrointest Tumors.* 2017; 3:125-7.

146 Larsson SC, Permert J, Håkansson N, Näslund I, Bergkvist L, Wolk A. Overall obesity, abdominal adiposity, diabetes and cigarette smoking in relation to the risk of pancreatic cancer in two Swedish population-based cohorts. *Br J Cancer.* 2005;93:1310-5.

147 Amling CL. Relationship between obesity and prostate cancer. *Curr Opin Urol.* 2005;15:167-71.

148 Parikesit D, Mochtar CA, Umbas R, Hamid AR. The impact of obesity towards prostate diseases. *Prostate Int.* 2016;4:1-6.

149 Stott-Miller M, Neuhouser ML, Stanford JL. Consumption of deep-fried foods and risk of prostate cancer. *Prostate.* 2013;73:960-9.

150 Touitou Y, Reinberg A, Touitou D. Association between light at night, melatonin secretion, sleep deprivation, and the internal clock: Health impacts and mechanisms of circadian disruption. *Life Sci.* 2017;173:94-106.

151 Stapleton JL, Tatum KL, Devine KA, Stephens S, Masterson M, Baig A, Hudson SV, Coups EJ. Skin Cancer Surveillance Behaviors Among Childhood Cancer Survivors. *Pediatr Blood Cancer.* 2016;63:554-7.

152 Tortorella SM, Royce SG, Licciardi PV, Karagiannis TC. Dietary Sulforaphane in Cancer Chemoprevention: The Role of Epigenetic Regulation and HDAC Inhibition. *Antioxid Redox Signal.* 2015;22:1382-424.

153 Bayat Mokhtari R, Baluch N, Homayouni TS, Morgatskaya E, Kumar S, Kazemi P, Yeger H. The role of Sulforaphane in cancer chemoprevention and health benefits: a mini-review. *J Cell Commun Signal.* 2018;121:91-101.

154 Egner PA, Chen JG, Zarth AT, Ng DK, Wang JB, Kensler KH, Jacobson LP, Muñoz A, Johnson JL, Groopman JD, Fahey JW, Talalay P, Zhu J, Chen TY, Qian GS, Carmella SG, Hecht SS, Kensler TW. Rapid and sustainable detoxication of airborne pollutants by broccoli sprout beverage: results of a randomized clinical trial in China. *Cancer Prev Res (Phila).* 2014;7:813-23.

155 Duthie SJ. Folate and cancer: how DNA damage, repair and methylation impact on colon carcinogenesis. *J Inherit Metab Dis.* 2011;34:101-9.

156 Bushman JL. Green tea and cancer in humans: a review of the literature. *Nutr Cancer.* 1998;31:151-9.

Abbreviations

in alphabetical

ACS	American Cancer Society
AGT	Angiotensinogen
AHA	American Heart Association
AHRQ	Agency for Healthcare Research and Quality
ALL	Acute lymphocytic leukemia
AML	Acute myeloid leukemia
Ang II	Angiotensin II
APM	Aspartame (L-aspartyl-L-phenylalanine methyl ester)
BHA	Butylated hydroxyanisole
BHT	Butylated hydroxytoluene
BMI	Body mass index
BPA	Bisphenol A
BPH	Benign prostatic hyperplasia
CO_2	Carbon dioxide
CDC	Centers for Disease Control and Prevention
CLL	Chronic lymphocytic leukemia
CML	Chronic myeloid leukemia
COPD	Chronic obstructive pulmonary disease
CRP	C-reactive protein

CT	Computed tomography
DASH	Dietary Approaches to Stop Hypertension
DNA	Deoxyribonucleic acid
DRE	Digital rectal exam
EBV	Epstein bar virus
EMFs	Electric and magnetic fields or electromagnetic fields
EPA	Environment Protection Agency
FAMMM	Familial atypical mole-malignant melanoma syndrome
FAP	Familial adenomatous polyposis
FCS	Fructose corn syrup
FDA	Food and Drug Administration
GMOs	Genetically modified organisms
GPR	G-protein-coupled receptor
HBOC	Hereditary breast-ovarian cancer
HCA	Heterocyclic amine
HDL	High density lipoprotein
HFCS	High-fructose corn syrup
HIV	Human immunodeficiency virus
HPV	Human papillomavirus
H. pylori	*Helicobacter pylori*
HRT	Hormone replacement therapy
IBD	Inflammatory bowel disease
IL	Interleukins
IL-6	Interleukine-6
IL-8	Interleukine-8
LAB	Lactic acid bacteria
IARC	International Agency for Research on Cancer
LDL	Low density lipoprotein

MRI	Magnetic resonance image
NIH	National Institute of Health
NO	Nitric oxide
NOCs	*N*-Nitroso compounds
OSA	Obstructive sleep apnea
PAD	Peripheral arterial disease or peripheral artery disease
PAH	Polycyclic aromatic hydrocarbon
PCE	Perchloroethylene
PSA	Prostate specific antigen
PUFA	n-3 polyunsaturated fatty acids
PVD	Peripheral vascular disease
RF	Radiofrequency
ROS	Reactive oxygen species
SAD	Standard American Diet
SAR	Specific absorption rate
SIDS	Sudden infant death syndrome
SPF	Sun protection factor
TB	Tuberculosis
TCM	Traditional Chinese medicine
TFA	Trans fatty acids
THC	Tetrahydrocannabinol
TNF-α	Tumor necrosis factor alpha
UV	Ultraviolet
VOCs	Volatile organic compounds
WHO	World Health Organization

Index

gut microbiota, 62–63, 182, 218–
219, 275

H

H. pylori (*Helicobacter pylori*), 104,
108, 196, 219
HDL (high-density lipoproteins), 26
head cancer, marijuana smoking
and, 156
healing energy, how to harness
in order to prevent cancer,
167–169
healthcare, embracing your role in,
288–290
healthspan, 127
healthy anticancer diet (HAD),
249–252
healthy habits, cultivation of, 129,
151, 202, 281–282
healthy lifestyle, with eco-friendly
actions, 85-86
heart disease. *See also* cardiovascular
disease
age and, 124–125
bad fats and, 24, 25, 27
BPA and, 39
chronic inflammation and, 117
climate change and, 85
hypertension and, 35
lead exposure and, 279
as leading killer of men and
women, 7, 26
obesity and, 56, 64, 68, 187
prevention of, 269, 272
SAD as linked to, 249
secondhand smoke as linked
to, 8, 9

sedentary lifestyle and, 46, 50,
51, 52
stress and, 140, 142
sugar consumption and, 30
Helicobacter pylori (H. pylori), 104,
108, 196, 219
heme iron, 21
hereditary breast-ovarian cancer
(HBOC), 218
hereditary melanoma, 92
heroin, 154, 155, 156
herpes virus type-8, 107. *See also*
KSHV
heterocyclic aromatic amines
(HCA), as carcinogen, 21,
22, 75, 209, 229
hexavalent chromium (Cr-6), as
carcinogen, 75
high blood pressure, 17, 35, 36, 45,
61, 64, 222, 241
high-density lipoproteins
(HDL), 26
high-fructose corn syrup (HFCS),
29, 30, 255
high-intensity interval training
(HIIT), 70
Hodgkin lymphoma
EBV as evident in, 107
HIV virus as participant in, 107
home, top cancer risks at, 77–79
hormonal factors, 22, 47, 55, 61, 64,
67, 70, 71, 118, 141, 142, 151,
165, 171, 172, 173, 174, 227
hormone replacement therapy
(HRT), and breast cancer
risk, 163, 170, 174
household cleaning products
and cancer-causing substances,
78–79

insomnia, 135
Institute of Medicine (IOM)
    on diagnostic error, 283
    on quality of care, 287
ionizing radiation, as carcinogen,
    98, 100, 196–197, 205, 236

K

kale, benefits of, 42, 73, 229, 247-
    248, 270
Kaposi sarcoma
    HIV virus as participant in, 107
    KSHV as cause of, 107
Kaposi sarcoma herpes virus
    (KSHV), 107
kidney cancer
    diabetes and, 34
    obesity and, 56, 61, 187
    steroid use and, 155
    tobacco smoking and, 6–7
    urinary tract infection and, 108

L

lactic acid bacteria (LAB), 274
Lao Tzu, 49
laughter, benefits of, 113, 127, 151
LDL (low-density lipoproteins), 26,
    58, 59
lead contamination, in water,
    278–280
learning, benefits of, 130
lemons, benefits of, 73
leukemia
    adult leukemia, 204–207
    childhood leukemia, 194–197
    risk and preventable factors of,
        204-205
liver cancer

aflatoxins and, 88–89
Hepatitis B virus and, 107
Hepatitis C virus and, 107
risk factors related, 6-7, 16, 40,
    61, 88-89, 107, 155, 156,
    157-158
longevity, traditional Chinese
    medicine (TCM) and, 125,
    127-130
love, benefits of, 130, 147, 291–292
low-density lipoproteins (LDL), 26,
    58, 59
lung cancer
    asbestos and, 256
    air pollution and, 88
    Chlamydia pneumoniae as
        linked to, 104
    marijuana smoking and, 156
    occupational link and
        protection, 212–214
    radon gas and, 78, **210-212**
    risk factors / key sources of,
        104, 208-212
    screening for, 214–215
    smoking and, 5, 7, 8, 77, 208–
        209, 230
lycopene, benefits of, 73, 97,
    228, 265
lymphoma. *See also* Hodgkin
    lymphoma; non-Hodgkin
    lymphoma
    as childhood cancer, 191
    EBV and, 107
    H. pylori and, 104
    KSHV as cause of, 107

324

M

magnetic resonance imaging (MRI), 60
malignancy, 2
mammogram, 169, 177, 286, 288
marijuana (or cannabis), and cancer risk, 154, 156–157
maternal smoking, impacts of on children, 9
meats. *See* processed meat; red meat
meditation, 126, 145, 151, 168, 261, 282
melanoma, 91, 92, 93, 175–176, 218, 233, 234, 235, 277–278
meridians, 125
metastasis, defined, 1
metastatic cancer, 1
mobile technology, cautions / safety, 101–103
monounsaturated fats, 24, 28
morphine, 155, 156
mutations
  acquired mutations, 2
  BRCA mutations, 166, 174, 175, 176
  genetic mutation, 2, 6, 131, 164, 183, 210, 218
  inherited mutations, 2, 131, 175

N

naphthalene, as possible human carcinogen, 76, 80
narcotic painkillers, 153, 155, 159
nasopharyngeal cancer
  Chinese style salted fish as associated with, 36
  EBV as case of, 107

National Cancer Institution, on alcohol intake, 18
neck cancer, marijuana smoking and, 156
Neisseria gonorrhoeae, as link to cancers, 105
NICE acronym, for monitoring physical and emotional wellness, 127–128
nicotine replacement therapy, 14, 15
nitric oxide (NO), 58, 61
nitrosamines, 21, 209, 218
non-Hodgkin lymphoma
  Hepatitis C virus and, 107
  HIV virus and, 107
  obesity and, 56, 187
  use of steroid, stimulants and, 155, 157
nonionizing radiation, 100, 103, 194
nuts and seeds, benefits of, 24, 73, 128, 229, 245, 247, 248, 250, 251, 267

O

oatmeal, benefits of, 72
obesity
  and aging, 62–63, 66-67
  and estrogen, 172-173
  bottleneck effect on weight gain, 65
  as chronic inflammatory disease, 118
  complexity of, 65–67
  defined, 56
  fat as involved in pathological changes, 58
  fat inside blood vessels, 59–60

qi gong, 126, 168

R

race and ethnicity, as uncontrollable
  risk factor for cancer, 131
radiation
  from cell phones, 90, 99–103,
    200, 230
  ionizing radiation, 98, 100,
    196–197, 205, 236
  as known risk factor for cancer,
    2, 90–103
  nonionizing radiation, 100,
    103, 194
  radiofrequency (RF) radiation,
    100–101, 193, 194, 200, 230
  ultraviolet (UV) radiation.
    See ultraviolet (UV)
    radiation
radiation therapy, 98, 197
radiofrequency (RF) radiation,
    100–101, 193, 194, 200, 230
radiofrequency electromagnetic
    fields, as possible human
    carcinogen, 100. *See also*
    electromagnetic fields
    (EMFs)
radon gas, as carcinogen, 77, 78, 79,
    196, 210, 211, 212, 213, 256
reactive oxygen species (ROS),
    17, 58, 59, 121, 137, 141,
    156–157
red meat
  as cancer risk, 219–220, 229
  as cause of cancer, 21–22, 75
  defined, 21
  as increasing colorectal cancer
    risk, 181

in SAD diet, 249
repetitive strength training, 54–55
resistance exercise (weight
    training), 54
resveratrol, benefits of, 97, 265
risk factors
  definition, 2
  for cancer. *See chapters 1-9,
    specific cancers*
ROOM acronym, for optimal sleep
    regimen, 138–139

S

SAD (standard American diet),
    249–252
salmon, benefits of, 24, 72, 97, 229,
    243, 246, 248, 250, 266
Salmonella species, and infection,
    105, 275–278
Salmonella typhi, 104
salt
  limiting intake of, 37–38
  link to hypertension and organ
    damage, 35–36
salty food, link to cancers, 36
SAR (specific absorption rate), 100
saturated fats, 22, 23, 24–25, 28,
    34, 115
screenings
  colonoscopy, 180, 184–185, 214
  genetic screening, 131, 169, 176
  for lung cancer, 214–215
  mammogram, 169, 177,
    286, 288
  for prostate cancer, 128, 214,
    227–228
  for skin cancer, 237

Printed in the United States
By Bookmasters